Vegan Bodybuilding Cookbook

100+ Tasty and Healthy Vegan Recipes To Improve Your Bodybuilding Training

Simon Arau

from various sources. Please consult a licensed professional before attempting any techniques outlined in this book.

By reading this document, the reader agrees that under no circumstances is the author responsible for any losses, direct or indirect, that are incurred as a result of the use of the information contained within this document, including, but not limited to, errors, omissions, or inaccuracies.

Table of Contents

Introduction

"The most ethical diet just so happens to be the most environmentally sound diet and just so happens to be the healthiest."

— Dr. Michael Greger

With so many diets to choose from and so much conflicting information out there, knowing what to eat has become more challenging than ever. And, as rates of chronic illness and obesity continue to rise, many are searching for a lifestyle that promotes overall good health. Veganism, not to be confused with vegetarian eating, has become more popular over the years. Veganism is the act of only consuming foods that are not associated with animals. Meat, dairy, eggs, and fish are not part of a vegan diet. Many vegans also do not eat honey or support brands that test on animals. However, because there are so many different reasons why people become vegan, some are left skeptical. Although different motivations resonate with different people, there are three primary reasons to embark on a vegan lifestyle.

Many choose to adopt a vegan diet for environmental reasons. With business focused marketing and propaganda, critical information has been pushed aside. Rainforest destruction, ocean dead zones, freshwater depletion, pollution, and world hunger are all huge issues linked to the animal production industry. In addition to environmental concerns, ethical motivations are also taken into account on a vegan diet. Many are unaware of the type of treatment animals endure for our satisfaction. Animals are being raised in less than desirable conditions, battling tons of illnesses, and are killed in inhumane ways—all to support the infrastructure of our country. Going vegan for yourself is also another great reason. Not only are you not supporting these things, but your body will become healthier as a result. Eating animal products has been linked to various conditions like diabetes, cardiovascular disease, certain cancers, and weight gain. This book will give scientific evidence supporting all of these claims.

Following an overview of the basics of veganism, this book will provide you with important information on nutrients—both macro and micro. Nutrients are important in any diet, because keeping the body healthy should always be the main goal. Consuming vitamins, minerals, fat, carbs, and protein is not only important for health reasons, but plays a huge factor in achieving your bodybuilding goals. This book will briefly explain what macronutrients and micronutrients are, and give helpful examples of each. In addition, we'll discuss what should be consumed and how much. You'll get a baseline on how to start eating the right amount of fats, proteins, and carbs to build a strong physique. When switching to a vegan diet, many are concerned with getting enough protein. However, consuming protein on a vegan bodybuilder's diet is simple, and after reading this book, your concerns will be dismissed.

You'll also find out more about some of the best vegan proteins available, with guidelines to help you know how much to consume. This section will also discuss calories and the specific numbers you should be taking in to meet your bodybuilding goals.

Once you have all of the information to get you started on your vegan bodybuilding journey, tons of recipes will be provided to guide you in your new lifestyle. Many of the recipes offer new takes on foods you already know and love. One of the best parts of being vegan is that most of the same foods can be enjoyed, but with modifications that support your health, the health of animals, and the health of the environment. Many recipes are developed with your busy lifestyle in mind. We understand you may not have a lot of time throughout your week. These recipes will give you an estimated preparation time and total time. Consider doubling recipes for meal prepping, or making enough to have leftovers throughout the week. Breakfast, lunch, dinner, and snack recipes will ensure you have plenty of meal options to choose from. Chapter 7 will also provide useful information surrounding what to eat before and after specific types of workouts.

After reading this book, you'll be prepared to not only start your vegan lifestyle, but also to work toward a healthy physique. This book is geared to bodybuilders, but offers useful information to help you achieve any desired healthy body type. If you're ready to become healthier inside and out—while building muscle—keep reading! Once you've finished, you can visit our website http://simonarau.me for additional information and bonus material.

Chapter 1:

No Meat, No Problem

First, let's gain a better understanding of the importance of cutting out animal products in daily life. Not only does the industry harm animals and the environment, but it is also harming your health. This chapter will provide easy-to-understand scientific research, clearly explaining some of the detrimental findings. After going through the basics of veganism, the chapter will move into what you should be eating. Fats, proteins, carbs, vitamins, and minerals will all be covered. You'll learn the importance of each, and find out what specific amounts are recommended for you. However, we'll maintain a focus on nutrients from a bodybuilder's perspective. These helpful tips will help you achieve your goals faster, all while promoting internal health. Keep in mind that when making large diet changes, it's best to consult with a physician first—especially if underlying suspected or diagnosed conditions are prevalent.

Why Vegan?

While the term "vegan" has become popular over the years, many are left feeling dubious whenever they hear the word. Many associate veganism with past millennial, Generation X health fads. While those fads may have been helpful and health oriented, the rise and fall of diets can be hard to keep up with. Diets and their popularity have come and gone. Trends regarding particular foods have even surfaced—kale, celery, and avocados may in fact be some of the trendiest foods on the market and in social media. While many don't doubt the health benefits these foods boast, the reputation of these items have been linked to unfavorable, hard to follow, young adult crazes. Many categorize veganism as simply another trend, or an ideal that is unattainable, though most would theoretically support saving animals and saving the planet all while becoming healthier at the same time. With so much information floating around, however, simple theories become clouded by propaganda and business-focused marketing.

In the United States, treating chronic diseases illnesses is a one-and-a-half trillion dollar industry according to the Milkin Study Institute (n.d.). We've all been told to "eat your fruits and vegetables"—it's a saying that's been around for ages. Well, your grandma and parents had the right idea. Because the vegan diet mainly consists of vegetables, fruits, whole grains, beans, legumes, and nuts, the amount of nutrients your body receives is drastically different than a meat heavy, processed diet. Consuming the right foods alone will ultimately lead to a better lifestyle and produce a desirable body. Even if you don't feel the immediate health effects after an unhealthy meal, there is still reason to eliminate animal products from your diet. According to a study by the Federal Commission for Nutrition (2015), meat is associated with an increased risk of total mortality, which takes into consideration the likelihood of developing diseases like cardiovascular disease, colorectal cancer, and type 2 diabetes. In fact, research has shown that processed meats like sausages, hot dogs, salami, ham, bacon, beef jerky, and canned meat can be classified as type one carcinogens—meaning there is sufficient evidence to link consumption of these meats with developing cancer (Q&A on the Carcinogenicity of the Consumption of Red Meat and Processed Meat, 2016). Scientific studies have shown clear links between meat and ill health, yet almost all food commercials on T.V. contain animal products. The research is out there, but is suppressed by the need to keep businesses like McDonald's, Burger King, and Taco Bell flourishing.

While many are aware of some of the studies surrounding beef specifically, it's important to know that chicken and dairy products are just as harmful. What many don't know is that the number one dietary source of cholesterol is chicken (Drewnowski & Rehm, 2013). This is because chicken are pumped full of sodium to ward off disease and infections picked up in their disgusting living quarters. With bacteria, fecal matter, and deceased chickens all in one space, it's not surprising chickens have to be given tons of antibiotics that you ultimately end up consuming. Dairy is similar in that it's not good for you. In simple terms, cow's milk is produced by a female cow and contains all the necessary ingredients to grow a baby cow. Like humans, babies need their mother's milk to survive. The only difference is, humans need human milk from their mothers. After consuming the life juice of a baby cow, it should come as no surprise that this contains elements that are unnatural and harmful to the human body. According to a study, for women who have had breast cancer, just one serving of dairy per day can increase their chances from dying from breast cancer by 49%, and dying from any disease by 64% (Kroenke et al, 2013). For men, eating dairy can increase their likelihood of getting prostate cancer by 34% (Prostate Cancer, n.d.).

In terms of the environment, producing large quantities of animal products has taken a detrimental toll. Raising, feeding, and keeping animals healthy enough for profit is an expensive endeavor on its own. According to the popular documentary *What the Health* (2017), raising animals for food is the leading cause for rainforest destruction (land), species extinction (loss of habitat), ocean dead zones (waste), and freshwater consumption degradation. Another huge problem looming in the environmental world is greenhouse gases and carbon emissions. You may be surprised to know that raising animals for consumption produces more greenhouse gases than the entire transportation sector (Key Facts and Findings, n.d.). This statistic takes into consideration the pollution given off by cars, trains, ships, airplanes, buses, and cargo ships. Greenhouse gases are associated with global warming or a changing of the Earth's natural processes, as proven by historical data. Here are a few more alarming statistics about the animal industry and its toll on the environment:

- A car would have to drive 200 miles to produce the same amount of emissions as one single burger containing half a pound of meat (Life-Cycle Analysis Study Suggests Eating Less Meat, 2019).

- Huge areas of rainforest are cleared for the supply of animal feed and for pasture land—the CO_2 emission soars to 335 kg for just one kilogram of beef (Life-Cycle Analysis Study Suggests Eating Less Meat, 2019).

- Studies show that going vegan can cut an individual's personal carbon footprint in half (New Study: Cut Your Carbon Footprint by Going Vegan, 2014).

- Humans produce enough grain to feed the world, but we choose to feed most of it to animals just so we can eat meat (Seufert, Ramankutty, & Foley, 2012).

- Animal agriculture is responsible for two-thirds of all freshwater consumption in the world today (Florio, 2015).

The last reason that many chose to go vegan is for ethical purposes. Cows, pigs, and chickens are all slaughtered for human consumption. In addition, many have a poor quality of life leading up to their death.

Comfort and cleanliness is thrown out the door by most businesses housing hundreds of animals for profit. These animals are constantly exposed to fecal matter and disease, but are continuously given medication to keep them well enough to be consumed by humans. However, according to Food Safety News (2010), "According to new data just released by the Food and Drug Administration (FDA), of the antibiotics sold in 2009 for both people and food animals, almost 80 percent were reserved for livestock and poultry." Keep in mind that the internal health of a chicken is not always visible, even on your dinner plate.

All About Nutrients: Macro & Micro

Macro and micro nutrients are similar in that the body needs both for optimal function. The difference lies with the amount the body requires daily. Macronutrients come from proteins, fats, and carbs, while micronutrients are found in vitamins and minerals. Macronutrients help the body run, while micronutrients keep the body in good health. The word *macro* means large. As you may know, your body relies on macronutrients for energy. Carbs and protein provide four calories per gram while fats provide nine calories per gram. Consuming all three macros in the right amounts will help you achieve your fitness goals.

If you're a bodybuilder or someone who dabbles in fitness, the word *protein* is likely very familiar. The Academy of Nutrition and Dietetics recommends that bodybuilders eat 1.2 to 1.7 grams of protein per kilogram (2.2 pounds) of body weight each day (Caspero, 2014). For example, a 190-pound bodybuilder should eat between 103 to 147 grams of protein daily. For some, consuming enough protein can be challenging. In theory, one could take their daily dose of protein in one sitting. However, this isn't recommended and could be dangerous. According to *Men's Health* (2019), the body can only absorb 25 to 35 grams of protein per sitting. Consuming protein throughout the day will keep the muscles strong and aid in recovery. The metabolism is like a fire that needs to be stoked every so often, but remember that throwing on a huge log may put it out. Protein intake should be divided up into meals and snacks, with an additional serving after a workout. For this example, an individual could consume 25 grams of protein at each meal, and 28 grams of protein after a workout. These numbers will be different for each person, but the bulk of your protein should come at meals and after workouts, with snacks in between.

Getting enough protein as a vegan is not as difficult as it seems. In fact, all protein is derived from plants—animal proteins originate from the plants they consumed (What About Protein: The Science on Protein, n.d.). Complete proteins are important for the body. A complete protein contains all of the nine essential amino acids. Because our body cannot produce all amino acids on its own, we must rely on food. While many animal proteins are considered to be complete proteins, other complications arise when consuming animal products. Because animals are the middleman when it comes to protein, plant protein is pure and delivers an abundance of nutrients. Luckily, many vegan foods contain complete proteins. Buckwheat, quinoa, and soy are a few examples. Eating certain foods in combination with others will also allow you to consume complete proteins. Rice and beans, Ezekiel bread, hummus and pita, and a peanut butter sandwich will provide complete proteins. Hemp and chia seeds are close to being complete proteins, but still give nutritional benefits regardless. Other proteins, though considered incomplete, still provide an array of nutrients. Although the body needs amino acids, the body also requires other nutrients that incomplete proteins contain. Other great vegan protein sources are lentils, beans, nutritional yeast, green peas, seitan, spirulina, oats, wild rice, and nuts. Many vegetables also aid in protein intake.

The second macronutrient is fat, which is imperative for energy, cellular health, insulation, absorbing nutrients, and regulating hormones. Fats have gained a negative reputation over the years. The truth is, not all fats are created equal and some fats should be avoided like the plague. The four types of fats are: saturated, monounsaturated, polyunsaturated, and trans. Monounsaturated and polyunsaturated fats are the healthiest and are found in foods like avocado, macadamia nuts, olives, walnuts, flax seeds, and brazil nuts. However, be aware that anything highly processed containing these fats should still be avoided. Monounsaturated fats protect the heart and support healthy insulin regulations. Polyunsaturated fats are important for receiving omega-3 and omega-6 fats, which reduce inflammation and regulate hormones.

The omegas also aid in the health of the brain, cells, and muscles. Saturated fats are mostly unhealthy, with a few exceptions. Vegans typically don't run into a problem with saturated fats, because most come from animal products. While the jury is still out on the importance of saturated fats, scientists do know that they're needed in small amounts, from healthy sources. Saturated fats, specifically from animals, are being investigated for possible links to many chronic illnesses. Because there are so many conflicting theories on saturated fats derived from animals, vegans can rest assured that the healthiest options are coconut oil and MCT oil. These saturated fats provide the body and brain with quick energy and raise the good HDL cholesterol in the blood. The last fat, trans fat, is undoubtedly the unhealthiest. Trans fats come from all processed and genetically modified foods. Corn, vegetable, and soy oils are examples of trans fats and are found in almost all "unhealthy" foods. Trans fats produce an inflammatory effect within the body and are believed to have links to other health complications.

Even through the body needs fats, fat is also helpful for bodybuilders looking to reach caloric goals. Fat contains twice the number of calories as carbs and proteins (per gram). According to *Healthline* (2019), the general recommendation for fat intake for an off-season bodybuilder is 1 gram per kg (0.5 grams per pound) of body weight. For example, an individual weighing 190 pounds should consume 95 grams of fat per day. Like protein, fat should be consumed throughout meals and not "taken" all at one time. It's recommended that no more than 60 grams of fat should be consumed in one sitting, as it puts high stress on the digestive system (Greenfield, 2017).

The third macronutrient is carbohydrates. Carbs are found in foods like fruits, vegetables, grains, nuts, legumes, seeds, and sweets, and are made of fiber, starch, and sugar. There are two types of carbs: simple and complex. Simple carbs give quick energy and are rapidly digested. A few examples of simple carbs are raw sugar, brown sugar, glucose, and fructose. Soda, baked treats, packaged sweets, and sugary cereals would be considered simple carbs. As you may know, these foods should be eaten in moderation or not at all, if working towards a fit physique. Simple carbs tend to be low in nutrition and might leave you with a headache if consumed in large amounts. On the other hand, complex carbs can be beneficial to achieving fitness goals. Complex carbs are typically high in fiber and digest slowly, giving long, sustained energy. Fruits, nuts, vegetables, beans, and whole grains all contain healthy carbohydrates. Be aware that even though the sugar found in complex carbs is generally healthy, you may want to monitor your intake for bodybuilding purposes. It's recommended that a high-endurance athlete should consume 2.3 to 5.5 grams of carbs per pound of body weight daily (Jeukendrup, 2011). For an individual weighing 190 pounds, this equates to 437 to 1,045 grams daily. Although this is a big range, the amount consumed should depend on how hard you're training and your fitness goals. Keep in mind that the harder the body trains, the more carbs it requires.

Calculating calories as a bodybuilder will be touch and go at first. Although there are general rules of thumb, everybody is different. The suggested amounts may need to be altered for you to achieve your goals, and will also depend on your gym schedule. *Science-MX Nutrition* (2019), a website for endurance trainers, suggests that a beginner would calculate calories by multiplying 20 calories per pound of body mass. A more advanced physique would multiply 25 calories per pound of body mass. Depending on your level and composition, this is a general place to start. Remember that the suggested macronutrients typically fall within a range, and can always be adjusted. However, you will see that the recommendations above will get you close to your caloric goals. We'll use the 190-pound individual as an example and take the medium amount for each recommendation above in regards to macronutrients. Remember that there are four calories per gram in protein/carbs and nine calories per gram of fat. If the 190-pound individual consumes 125 grams of protein, 95 grams of fat, and 741 grams of carbs, 4,319 calories have been consumed. This caloric intake would fall in line with the suggested amount.

Micronutrients are different from macronutrients specifically in regards to the quantity needed by the body. Micronutrients are vitamins and minerals. Vitamins are used for energy, immune health, blood clotting, and other important basic functions. Minerals keep bones healthy, aid in growth, regulate fluids, and keep the body strong. Vitamins are derived from plants, while minerals are derived from soil and water. There are four types of micronutrients: water-soluble, fat-soluble, macrominerals, and trace minerals.

Water-soluble vitamins are able to dissolve when placed into water, meaning the water is a carrier. Water-soluble vitamins aren't typically stored in the body and are flushed out during urination. Popular water-soluble vitamins include biotin, folate, thiamine, and riboflavin, which are all apart of the B-vitamin group. Vitamin C is also considered a water-soluble vitamin. These vitamins are essential for energy, cell function, metabolization of foods, and blood health.

Fat-soluble vitamins do not dissolve in water and are best absorbed when consumed with a source of fat. Fat-soluble vitamins are stored in the liver and fatty tissues for future use. Fat-soluble vitamins include vitamin A, vitamin D, vitamin E, and vitamin K. Their roles in the body deal with vision health, organ function, immune health, bone growth, protecting cells, and blood clotting.

Macrominerals are needed in larger amounts than trace minerals, thus giving them the name macro. Macrominerals include calcium, phosphorus, magnesium, sodium, chloride, potassium, and sulfur. Their duties range from bone structure, blood vessel health, aiding in enzyme reactions, regulating blood pressure, maintaining hydration, regulating fluids, to the actual structure of the body.

Lastly, trace minerals include iron, manganese, copper, iodine, fluoride, selenium, and zinc. Trace minerals are needed in smaller amounts but still are important for providing oxygen to muscles, creating certain hormones, assisting in metabolization, tissue health, brain health, nervous system health, and wound healing.

Overall, micronutrients are an essential part of the diet for basic human health. Your body needs micronutrients to even function. Luckily, the vegan diet contains many healthy foods, and eating a variety of fruits, vegetables, nuts, beans, legumes, and seeds will help you get all the micronutrients you need. Vitamins and minerals can also act as antioxidants, which may protect against cell damage associated with diseases like cancer, Alzheimer's, and heart disease (Streit, 2018).

Chapter 2:

Breakfast

This section will take you through recipes for breakfast. Each recipe explains how much time is needed, serving size, and nutritional information. Keep in mind that some of the nutritional information will depend on the products used. Many of these recipes can be mixed and matched. Every recipe is 100% vegan and plant based, and many are modern takes on foods you may already love. One of the best things about going vegan is that almost all of the same foods can be enjoyed—with a much higher nutritional value. While most if not all the recipes are healthy, you can make small adjustments to increase protein, lower calories, add fats, etc. You may not have time to make different recipes throughout the entire week, so it's suggested you increase or reduce the servings depending on the size of your family.

Breakfast Recipe: One

Breakfast Burrito or Bowl

Nutritional Information Per Serving: 183 calories, 5 grams fat, 6 grams fiber, 17 grams protein, 20 grams carbs

Time: 35 minutes

Serving Size: 4 servings

Ingredients:

- 14 ounces (one package) tofu, extra firm
- 1 teaspoon of olive oil
- 3 teaspoons garlic, minced
- 1 medium onion, diced
- 1 cup potato, diced
- 1½ cup mushrooms, sliced
- ¼ cup nutritional yeast
- 3 tablespoons fresh basil, minced
- 2 tablespoons parsley
- 1 tablespoon fresh lemon juice
- Himalayan salt and black pepper to preference

*Optional: whole grain tortillas of choice, salsa, vegan cheese, guacamole, hot sauce, etc.

Directions:

1. Rinse the tofu and press firmly to remove as much water as possible. Use clean kitchen towels if necessary.

2. In a large skillet, add oil, garlic, and onion over medium heat. Stir occasionally until the onions are translucent and soft.

3. Add potatoes and mushrooms to skillet and sauté for 10 minutes. Stir frequently to avoid burning.

4. Add the tofu to the skillet and use a spatula to mash the tofu into very small pieces.

5. Reduce the heat to a low simmer and add in nutritional yeast, herbs, lemon juice, Himalayan salt, and black pepper.

6. Continue to let the mixture cook until potatoes are soft, then remove the skillet from heat.

7. Serve the mixture warm or on a tortilla with desired vegan toppings.

Breakfast Recipe: Two

Casserole Strata

Nutritional Information Per Serving: 348 calories, 14 grams fat, 5 grams fiber, 11 grams protein, 49 grams carbs

Time: 30 minutes prep, 1 hour 20 minutes total

Serving Size: 6 servings

Ingredients:

- 2 medium zucchini, sliced into thin rings
- 1 medium tomato, drained and diced
- 1 medium onion, finely chopped
- 4 cloves garlic, crushed
- 1 teaspoon Italian seasoning
- 1 tablespoons avocado oil
- 1 tablespoon olive oil
- 1 jalapeño, finely chopped
- 10 basil leaves (for garnish)
- 4 leaves sage, minced
- 1 cup cashews
- ½ lemon, juiced
- 4 potatoes, peeled
- 5 slices sourdough bread, sliced into cubes
- Himalayan salt and black pepper to preference

Directions:

1. Place cashews in a bowl and pour hot water over the top. Set aside, and allow the cashews to soak for 30 minutes.
2. Preheat the oven to 350°F and set aside a 9 x 12 inch baking pan.
3. In a pot, boil the peeled potatoes until soft. Remove from heat when finished.
4. In a skillet, warm the avocado oil and add the garlic over medium heat.
5. Quickly add in zucchini, tomatoes, onions, black pepper, and Italian seasoning. Stir frequently to avoid burning.
6. Sauté for 5 minutes or until the zucchini is soft, but not mushy. No liquid should remain in the pan, so drain if necessary. Remove from heat.
7. Drain the cashews and place cashews, 2 cups of water, basil, lemon juice, salt, and jalapeño in a blender. Blend until smooth and creamy. Add Himalayan salt to your preference.
8. When the potatoes are soft, mash them and add in olive oil, Himalayan salt, and sage. You can mash the potatoes by hand or using a blender, but the consistency should remain thick.
9. In a large bowl, mix the zucchini and tomato mixture along with the cubed breadcrumbs. Add in half of the potatoes and stir.

10. Add the mixture evenly to a 9 x 12 inch baking dish.

11. Pour cashew sauce over the top of the mixture and press down using a spatula to gently soak the bread.

12. Add the remaining potatoes to the top.

13. Place the dish into the oven and bake for 40 minutes.

14. After 40 minutes has passed, use the broiler feature on the oven and broil until the top is golden brown. This should take anywhere from 5 to 10 minutes.

15. Remove the casserole from the oven and garnish with basil. Serve warm.

Breakfast Recipe: Three

Avocado Toast

Nutritional Information Per Serving: 665 calories, 47 grams fat, 25 grams fiber, 21 grams protein, 54 grams carbs

Time: 10 minutes

Serving Size: 1 serving

Ingredients:

- 2 slices of Ezekiel Bread, toasted (another hearty, seeded bread can be substituted)
- 1 ripe avocado, pitted
- 2 tablespoons pepitas
- 1 tablespoon chia seeds
- 1 tablespoon hemp seeds
- ¼ whole lemon
- Himalayan salt and black pepper to preference

Directions:

1. In a bowl, add avocado, salt, pepper, chia seeds, and hemp seeds.
2. Evenly spread the mixture over the toasted bread.

3. Sprinkle with pepitas.
4. Squeeze the lemon over the top to finish.

Breakfast Recipe: Four

Vegetable Omelet

Nutritional Information Per Serving: 590 calories, 32 grams fat, 12 grams fiber, 22 grams protein, 52 grams carbs

Time: 20 minutes

Serving Size: 1 serving (yields 2 omelettes)

Ingredients:

- ¼ cup chickpea flour
- ⅔ cup water
- 2 tablespoon nutritional yeast
- 2 tablespoon avocado oil
- ½ cup veggies of choice, diced
- Himalayan salt and black pepper to preference

Directions:

1. In a bowl, mix chickpea flour, nutritional yeast, salt, and water. Stir until no lumps remain.
2. Add half of the oil to a non-stick frying pan and sauté the vegetables over low heat until tender. Add the vegetables to the batter and mix well.

3. Increase heat to medium, and pour half of the batter into the frying pan.
4. Cook for 5 minutes and flip. This procedure is similar to when making pancakes.
5. Cook for an additional 3 to 5 minutes or until the middle is no longer soft.
6. Repeat steps 2 through 5 to cook the second omelette. Use a dash of oil as needed to prevent burning.

Breakfast Recipe: Five

Breakfast Sandwich

Nutritional Information Per Serving: 573 calories, 30 grams fat, 7 grams fiber, 30 grams protein, 54 grams carbs

Time: 15 minutes

Serving Size: 2 servings

Ingredients:

- 3 tablespoons soy sauce
- 1½ tablespoons maple syrup
- 1 tablespoon apple cider vinegar
- 1 teaspoon garlic, minced
- 1 teaspoon smoked paprika
- 8 ounce package tempeh
- 1 tablespoon olive oil
- 2 or 3 vegan english muffins (substitute for bread if necessary)
- ½ avocado, pitted and sliced
- ½ cup arugula (substitute spinach if necessary)
- Himalayan salt and black pepper to preference
- sauce of choice (ketchup, mustard, vegan mayo, etc.)

Directions:

1. In a small bowl, whisk together soy sauce, maple syrup, apple cider vinegar, garlic, paprika, and black pepper.
2. Slice the tempeh in half. Then slice each section again, and again. You will end up with 6 slabs total.
3. In a large skillet, add olive oil and turn the stove to medium-high heat.
4. Place the tempeh slabs into the pan evenly to brown the bottoms. Brown for about 3 minutes.
5. Pour the sauce over the tempeh, into the skillet.
6. Flip the tempeh and cook for an additional 3 minutes. Most of the liquid should be absorbed and both sides of the tempeh browned.
7. Prepare the english muffins by toasting and adding on the tempeh. Add all other toppings and your desired sauce.

Breakfast Recipe: Six

Tofu Quiche

Nutritional Information Per Serving: 178 calories, 9 grams fat, 4 grams fiber, 7 grams protein, 20 grams carbs

Time: 15 minutes prep, 1 hour and 45 minutes total

Serving Size: 8 servings

Ingredients:

For the crust:
- 3 large potatoes
- 2 tablespoons olive oil
- ¼ teaspoon sea salt
- ¼ teaspoon pepper

For the filling:
- 12.3 ounces silken tofu, extra firm
- 2 tablespoons nutritional yeast
- 3 tablespoons hummus
- 3 garlic cloves, roughly chopped
- 1 medium onion, diced
- ¾ cup cherry tomatoes, halved
- 1 cup broccoli, roughly chopped

- sea salt and pepper to preference

Directions:

1. Remove tofu from the package and press using clean dish towels. Remove as much moisture as possible and set aside.
2. Preheat the oven to 450°F. Lightly coat a 9.5-inch pie pan with non-stick spray or a dab of oil.
3. Grate the potatoes and measure out 3 cups. Transfer the shreds to a clean dish towel and squeeze out as much water as possible.
4. Add the potato shreds to a pie dish and drizzle with olive oil. Toss in salt and pepper.
5. Using your fingers, press the potato into the pan and up the sides to form an even layer. This will serve as the crust of the quiche.
6. Set the pie pan in the oven for 30 minutes or until crust is golden brown all over. Set the pie aside.
7. Turn the oven to 400°F.
8. While the pie crust is cooking, prepare the vegetables by chopping and tossing with olive oil, salt, pepper, or any other desired spices.
9. Line a baking sheet with parchment paper and roast the vegetables for 20 or 30 minutes until soft and crispy. Remove and set aside.

10. Afterwards, lower the oven temperature to 375°F.

11. While the vegetables are cooking, prepare the tofu filling by adding it to a food processor with nutritional yeast, hummus, salt, and black pepper. Blend until smooth.

12. To assemble the quiche, remove the vegetables from the oven when finished and place them in a mixing bowl. Mix in the tofu mixture. Stir well to make sure the vegetables are evenly coated.

13. Add the mixture into the pie, smoothing out the top to make an even layer.

14. Bake the quiche for 30 to 40 minutes until the top appears firm and golden.

15. Serve warm and top with fresh herbs, green onion, or hot sauce if desired.

Breakfast Recipe: Seven

Protein Muffins

Nutritional Information Per Serving (1 muffin): 94 calories, 4 grams fat, 2 grams fiber, 8.6 grams protein, 6 grams carbs

Time: 15 minutes prep, 55 minutes total

Serving Size: 6 muffins

Ingredients:

- 15 ounces tofu (one package), medium firm
- 2 teaspoons tahini
- 2 tablespoons chickpea flour
- 3 tablespoons nutritional yeast
- 1 tablespoon miso paste
- ¼ teaspoon turmeric
- ½ teaspoon onion powder
- ½ teaspoon cayenne pepper flakes (optional)
- 3 cloves garlic, finely chopped
- 1 cup broccoli, roughly chopped
- 1 red bell pepper, diced
- ½ cup corn, drained and rinsed
- 2 scallions, roughly chopped
- Himalayan salt and black pepper to preference

Directions:

1. Preheat oven to 350°F. Line a muffin tin with six liners or lightly coat with non-stick spray.
2. In a skillet, add the garlic cloves and oil. Simmer over high heat for a minute before reducing to medium heat.
3. Add in the broccoli, bell pepper, corn, salt, and pepper to the skillet. Sauté for 2 minutes and remove from heat. The vegetables will be thoroughly cooked in the oven later.
4. Add the chopped scallion to the vegetables.
5. Place tofu in a food processor and puree until smooth.
6. Add chickpea flour, nutritional yeast, tahini, miso paste, turmeric, onion powder, salt, and pepper to the food processor. Continue to puree until smooth.
7. Combine the vegetables and tofu mixture. Mix well.
8. Distribute the batter evenly among the six muffin tins.
9. Bake for 25 to 35 minutes until the tops are lightly browned, rotating the muffin pan as necessary.
10. Remove from oven and allow the muffins to cool on a rack for 10 minutes before serving.

Breakfast Recipe: Eight

Protein Packed Chorizo

Nutritional Information Per Serving: 210 calories, 4 grams fat, 12 grams protein, 6 grams fiber, 32 grams carbs

Time: 25 minutes

Serving Size: 4 servings

Ingredients:

- ½ yellow onion, chopped into bite-sized chunks
- 1 cup red lentils, dry
- 2 cups vegetable broth
- 2 tablespoons apple cider vinegar
- 1 tablespoon olive oil

Suggested seasonings:
- 1 tablespoon cumin seed
- 1 tablespoon garlic powder
- 1 tablespoon smoked paprika
- 1 teaspoon coriander seed
- ½ teaspoon cumin
- ¼ teaspoon ground bay leaves
- ¼ teaspoon ground oregano
- ¼ teaspoon thyme

- sea salt and black pepper to preference

Directions:

1. Place lentils into a saucepan with 2 cups of vegetable broth. Bring to a boil before reducing to low heat. Cook the lentils for 10 to 15 minutes or until no liquid remains.
2. Add cumin seed and coriander seed to a small saucepan. Over medium heat, toast the seeds for 10 minutes. Stir occasionally to prevent burning.
3. In a separate, medium-sized saucepan, add oil and onions. Sauté for 6 minutes before adding all suggested spices. Stir and mix well.
4. When the cumin and coriander seeds are toasted and aromatic, crush them using a mortar pestle or with a blender. Add them to the onions.
5. When the lentils are finished, add them to the same pan as the onions and cook for 3 minutes to integrate all the flavors. The mixture should be quite dry and crumbly when finished.
6. Serve the chorizo over other breakfast recipes to add extra flavor and protein to meals.

Breakfast Recipe: Nine

Hummus Toast

Nutritional Information Per Serving: 316 calories, 16 grams fat, 19 grams protein, 14 grams fiber, 24 grams carbs

Time: 5 minutes

Serving Size: 1 serving

Ingredients:

- 2 slices sprouted/seeded grain wheat bread
- ¼ cup hummus (any flavor)
- 1 tablespoon hemp seeds
- 1 tablespoons roasted sunflower seeds
- ¼ teaspoon smoked paprika powder
- ¼ lemon (optional)
- black pepper to preference

Directions:

1. Place bread in the toaster.
2. Assemble the toast by smearing hummus evenly onto each slice.
3. Sprinkle with hemp seeds, sunflower seeds, paprika, and black pepper.

4. Squeeze lemon juice over the top to finish.

Breakfast Recipe: Ten

Classic Breakfast

Nutritional Information Per Serving: 735 calories, 36 grams fat, 37 grams protein, 22 grams fiber, 74 grams carbs

Time: 10 minutes prep, 20 minutes total

Serving Size: 1 serving

Ingredients:

For the English muffin:
- ⅓ cup rolled oats
- 1 tablespoon of chia seeds
- 2 tablespoons applesauce, unsweetened
- ½ teaspoon baking powder
- 1 tablespoon almond milk, unsweetened

For the eggs:
- ½ tablespoon olive oil
- 8 ounces (½ package) tofu, extra firm
- 1 tablespoon nutritional yeast
- ⅛ teaspoon turmeric
- 1 tablespoon almond milk
- Himalayan salt and black pepper to preference

For the sides:

- ½ avocado, pitted and sliced
- ½ medium tomatoes, sliced
- ½ cup baked beans, vegetarian

Directions:

1. To prepare the English muffin, add oats, chia seeds, and baking powder to a blender. Blend for 1 minute. Transfer the mixture into a bowl when finished.
2. Add applesauce and almond milk to the bowl. Stir until a dough forms.
3. Using your hands, flatten the dough into the shape of an English muffin and return it to the bowl.
4. Microwave for 2 minutes and 15 seconds. Then remove the bowl from the microwave and let the muffin rest for 5 minutes.
5. To prepare the eggs, heat the olive oil over medium heat in a skillet for 30 seconds.
6. Using your hands, crumble the tofu directly into the skillet. Mash further using a fork. Cook for 4 minutes until no water remains.
7. Add nutritional yeast, salt, pepper, and turmeric into the skillet. Stir constantly for 5 minutes.
8. Pour the almond milk into the skillet and stir. Turn the heat off and set eggs aside until ready to be served.

9. Prepare the breakfast plate by warming baked beans, slicing the tomato, and preparing the avocado.

10. Slice the English muffin in half and serve with any additional vegan sauces or toppings.

Breakfast Recipe: Eleven

Smoothie Bowl

Nutritional Information Per Serving: 550 calories, 23 grams fat, 26 grams protein, 16 grams fiber, 68 grams carbs

Time: 5 minutes

Serving Size: 1 serving

Ingredients:

For the smoothie:
- 1 large banana, frozen
- ½ cup almond milk (chocolate or vanilla)
- 1 scoop vegan protein powder (flavor of choice)
- 1 cup spinach
- handful of ice cubes

For the toppings:
- 1 tablespoon almond butter, melted
- 1 tablespoon of chia seeds
- ½ cup blueberries (or berries of choice)
- 2 tablespoons coconut flakes, unsweetened

Directions:

1. Add all smoothie ingredients to a blender and
    blend until smooth. The consistency should be
    thick, so do not add too much almond milk or
    ice.
2. Pour the smoothie into a large bowl.
3. Sprinkle desired toppings over the bowl. Enjoy
    immediately.

Breakfast Recipe: Twelve

Cinnamon & Apple Quinoa

Nutritional Information Per Serving: 372 calories, 10 grams fat, 8 grams fiber, 9 grams protein, 65 grams carbs

Time: 30 minutes

Serving Size: 2 servings

Ingredients:

- ½ cup quinoa
- 1 ½ cup water
- 2 large apples
- 2 teaspoons cinnamon
- ¼ cup sliced almonds

Directions:

1. Wash both apples. Peel and core the apples before chopping them into small pieces.
2. In a saucepan, add quinoa and apples. Bring the water to a boil before reducing to a simmer. Allow the quinoa and apples to simmer for 20 to 25 minutes. The apples should be soft and little to no water should remain.

3. Stir in the cinnamon and mix well.

4. Transfer the quinoa to a bowl and sprinkle almonds, additional cinnamon, or any other desired toppings.

Breakfast Recipe: Thirteen

Blueberry Baked Oatmeal

Nutritional Information Per Serving: 426 calories, 16 grams fat, 10 grams fiber, 14 grams protein, 61 grams carbs

Time: 15 minutes prep, 50 minutes total

Serving Size: 4 servings

Ingredients:

- 2 cups oats
- 2 cups water, boiling hot
- 2½ large bananas
- 1 flax egg (1 tablespoon ground flaxseed, 3 tablespoons water)
- ¼ cup maple syrup
- ¼ cup protein powder of choice
- ¼ cup hemp seeds
- ½ cup blueberries
- ¼ cup sliced almonds
- 2 teaspoons nutmeg
- 1 teaspoon cinnamon
- 1 teaspoon vanilla extract
- 1½ cups coconut milk (can substitute with almond, or other plant milk)

Directions:

1. Prepare the flax egg by mixing the ground flax and water. Stir well and place in the refrigerator for at least 15 minutes to thicken.
2. Preheat oven to 350°F. Set aside a 9 x 13 inch baking pan.
3. In a mixing bowl, add the oats and boiling water. Allow the oats to soak for 15 minutes.
4. In a separate bowl, take 2 bananas and mash until smooth. Stir in the flax egg, maple syrup, and protein powder. Mix well.
5. Add the banana mixture to the oats, and combine.
6. Stir in remaining ingredients, excluding the ½ banana.
7. Pour the oat mixture into the baking pan. Slice the remaining ½ banana for topping.
8. Bake for 30 to 35 minutes.
9. Remove and allow cooling before serving. Other toppings such as almond butter, nuts, or additional berries can be used for extra protein/nutrients if desired.

Breakfast Recipe: Fourteen

Pancakes

Nutritional Information Per Pancake: 151 calories, 8 grams fat, 2 grams fiber, 3 grams protein, 14 grams carbs

Time: 25 minutes

Serving Size: 10 pancakes

Ingredients:

- 2 tablespoons flaxseed meal
- 6 tablespoons water
- 1 cup quinoa flour
- ½ cup almond flour
- 2 teaspoons of coconut flour
- 2 teaspoons baking powder
- 1¼ cup coconut milk
- 3 tablespoons coconut oil, melted
- 1 tablespoon maple syrup
- 1 cup blueberries or ½ cup vegan chocolate chips
- pinch of Himalayan salt

Directions:

1. Prepare the flax egg by beating water with ground flax. Set this in the refrigerator for at least 15 minutes.
2. In a large bowl, whisk together all flours, baking powder, and salt.
3. In a separate bowl, beat the flax egg, milk, oil, and syrup.
4. Slowly combine the wet and dry mixtures. Stir well to form a smooth batter.
5. Fold in blueberries or chocolate chips.
6. Heat a griddle or non-stick pan over medium heat. Lightly spray with cooking oil or use a dab of coconut oil to grease the pan.
7. Ladle ¼ cup of batter per one pancake. Cook each pancake for 2 to 3 minutes, until small bubbles form around the edges.
8. Flip the pancakes and cook on the opposite side for an additional 1 or 2 minutes. The sides should look golden brown.
9. Serve warm and top with desired toppings such as maple syrup, nut butter, or fruit.

Breakfast Recipe: Fifteen

Breakfast Bars

Nutritional Information Per Serving: 446 calories, 16 grams fat, 10 grams fiber, 14 grams protein, 65 grams carbs

Time: 10 minutes prep, 35 minutes total

Serving Size: 12 bars, 6 servings

Ingredients:

- 1¼ cups oats, dry
- 1 cup quinoa, cooked
- ¼ cup coconut sugar
- 1 teaspoon baking powder
- 2 tablespoons ground flaxseed
- 6 tablespoons water
- 2 medium bananas
- ¼ cup almond butter
- 1 tablespoon vanilla extract
- ½ cup coconut flakes
- ¼ cup vegan chocolate chips
- pinch of Himalayan salt

Directions:

1. Prepare the flax egg by whisking water and the ground flax. Place in the refrigerator for at least 15 minutes.
2. Preheat the oven to 350°F. Line a 9-inch baking pan with parchment paper.
3. In a large bowl, mix together oats, quinoa, sugar, salt, and baking powder.
4. Remove the flax egg from the refrigerator and beat in banana, almond butter, and vanilla.
5. Slowly combine the dry and wet ingredients.
6. Fold in coconut flakes and chocolate chips to the mixture.
7. Pour batter into the baking pan evenly. Bake for 20 to 25 minutes until the top is golden brown.
8. Allow to cool before slicing into 12 portions. Store the bars in an airtight container in the refrigerator or pantry.

Breakfast Recipe: Sixteen

High-Protein, Muscle-Building Smoothie

Nutritional Information Per Serving: 945 calories, 28 grams fat, 34 grams fiber, 38 grams protein, 150 grams carbs

Time: 6 minutes

Serving Size: 1 serving

Ingredients:

- 2 bananas
- 1 cup plant milk (coconut, almond, oat, soy, etc.)
- 2 cups fresh spinach leaves
- ½ teaspoon turmeric
- pinch of black pepper
- 3 tablespoons chia seeds
- 1 teaspoon peanut butter
- ½ cup chickpeas
- 2 tablespoons dried dates
- water/ice (as needed)

Directions:

1. In a high-speed blender, add all ingredients. Pulse a few times before turning to the blend feature.
2. Add water and ice as needed to reach desired consistency.

Breakfast Recipe: Seventeen

Quick Oatmeal

Nutritional Information Per Serving: 620 calories, 21 grams fat, 13 grams fiber, 21 grams protein, 94 grams carbs

Time: 7 minutes

Serving Size: 1 serving

Ingredients:

- 2 cups instant/quick oatmeal, cooked
- 1 tablespoon maple syrup
- 1 medium banana
- 2 tablespoons hemp seeds
- 1 tablespoon almond butter

Directions:

1. Assemble the oatmeal by combining the cooked oats and maple syrup.
2. Top with sliced banana, almond butter, and hemp seeds.
3. Serve warm or cold.

Breakfast Recipe: Eighteen

Peanut Butter Pudding

Nutritional Information Per Serving: 300 calories, 16 grams fat, 4 grams fiber, 10 grams protein, 27 grams carbs

Time: 7 minutes

Serving Size: 6 servings

Ingredients:

- 28 ounces (2 packages) tofu, extra firm
- ½ cup oat milk
- ¾ cup peanut butter
- ½ cup cocoa powder, unsweetened
- 7 tablespoons honey
- 1 medium banana

Directions:

1. Remove tofu from packaging and wrap tofu in a clean dish towel. Place the tofu between two large plates. Set a heavy bowl on top to press down on the tofu. Leave the tofu for 5 minutes. The goal is to remove as much water as possible.

2. Add plant milk, peanut butter, cocoa powder, honey, and tofu to a high-speed blender. Blend for a few minutes until the pudding has reached a smooth consistency.

3. Top with desired toppings such as sliced banana or nuts. Store in the refrigerator, covered.

Breakfast Recipe: Nineteen

Protein Cookies

Nutritional Information Per Cookie: 100 calories, 2.8 grams fat, 2.5 grams fiber, 5.2 grams protein, 9 grams carbs

Time: 25 minutes

Serving Size: 6 cookies

Ingredients:

- 1½ medium banana, ripe
- ¼ cup sunflower seeds, unsalted
- 2 teaspoons of chia seeds
- ¼ cup flax meal
- 1 tablespoon almond flour
- 1 cup vegan, vanilla protein powder
- 2 tablespoons vegan chocolate chips

Directions:

1. Preheat oven to 350°F. Line a baking sheet with parchment paper.
2. In a bowl, mash bananas using a fork. The consistency should be as smooth as possible with no lumps.

3. Add chia seeds and ground flax to the bowl containing the mashed bananas. Mix until well combined.

4. Add in protein powder, peanut flour, and chocolate chips. Stir well but do not over process, as the batter can become too firm.

5. Using your hands or an ice cream scooper, split the batter into 6 equal cookies. Use your palm to roll the batter into ball.

6. Place the cookie balls onto the baking sheet and press down.

7. Bake for 8 minutes or until edges are golden brown.

8. Remove cookies and place onto a cooling rack for at least 10 minutes before consuming.

Breakfast Recipe: Twenty

Granola

Nutritional Information Per Serving: 240 calories, 10 grams fat, 7.5 grams protein, 5 grams fiber, 31 grams carbs

Time: 5 minutes prep, 35 minutes total

Serving Size: 16 servings (per ⅓ cup)

Ingredients:

- 3 cups old-fashioned oats
- 1 cup pecans
- ½ cup pepitas
- ½ cup sunflower seeds, salted
- ½ cup coconut flakes
- 1 teaspoon pumpkin pie spice
- ⅔ cup maple syrup
- ½ cup 100% pumpkin puree
- 1 teaspoon vanilla extract

Directions:

1. Preheat the oven to 300°F. Line a baking sheet with parchment paper.

2. In a bowl, mix oats, pecans, pepitas, sunflower seeds, coconut flakes, and spices.
3. In a separate bowl, whisk together pumpkin puree and maple syrup.
4. Combine the dry and wet ingredients. Stir until everything is evenly coated.
5. Spread the mixture on the baking sheet and bake for 45 minutes. Stir halfway though.
6. Remove granola and allow cooling before transferring it to an airtight container.

Chapter 3:

Lunch

This section will take you through recipes for lunch. Many of the recipes range from light to filling. Whether you prefer a big breakfast or wait until lunch for a larger meal, this chapter will include recipes for both situations. If you are not a fan of some of the ingredients, remember that nuts, vegetables, fruits, and sauces can all be interchanged. Each recipe can be adjusted into something you'll love!

Lunch Recipe: One

The Ultimate Chili

Nutritional Information Per Serving: 390 calories, 1 grams fat, 26 grams protein, 22 grams fiber, 65 grams carbs

Time: 10 minutes prep, 40 minutes total

Serving Size: 6 servings

Ingredients:

For the crumbles:
- 2 tablespoons soy sauce
- 2 tablespoons nutritional yeast
- 2 teaspoons chili powder
- 1 teaspoon smoked paprika
- 14 ounces (1 package) tofu, firm

For the chili:
- 1 medium onion, diced
- 3 garlic cloves, minced
- 56 ounces (2 cans) crushed tomatoes
- 30 ounces (2 cans) black beans, drained and rinsed

- 15 ounces (1 can) kidney beans, drained and rinsed
- 1 cup water
- 3 tablespoons chili powder
- 2 teaspoons ground cumin
- 1 tablespoon maple syrup
- 1 tablespoon cocoa powder
- 1 teaspoon smoked paprika
- ¼ teaspoon cayenne pepper (optional)
- Himalayan salt and black pepper to preference

Directions:

1. Preheat oven to 350°F. Line a baking sheet with parchment paper.
2. To make the tofu crumbles, mix soy sauce, nutritional yeast, chili powder, and smoked paprika in a medium-sized bowl.
3. Using your hands, crumble the tofu into the spices. Mix using hands or a spoon until mixture is combined evenly.
4. Spread the tofu mixture onto the baking sheet and bake for 30 minutes. Stir the tofu halfway through.
5. While the tofu is cooking, add a few drops of water, onion, and garlic to a large pot over medium heat. Stir frequently and simmer for 4

minutes. Use water as needed to prevent burning.

6. Add all other chili ingredients to the pot and mix well.
7. Bring chili to boil before reducing to low heat. Allow the chili to simmer for 20 minutes (the tofu should be complete after this time). Stir the chili occasionally.
8. Remove the tofu crumbles from the oven when finished, and add them to the chili.
9. Allow the chili to simmer for an additional 5 minutes. Serve with other vegan toppings of your choice such as cilantro, tortilla chips, tomatoes, avocado, chives, hot sauce, or vegan cheese.

Lunch Recipe: Two

Carnitas

Nutritional Information Per Serving: 145 calories, 11 grams fat, 1 gram protein, 1 grams fiber, 12 grams carbs

Time: 10 minutes prep, 50 minutes total

Serving Size: 4 servings

Ingredients:

- 1 tablespoon avocado oil
- ½ red onion, diced
- 40 ounces (2 cans) young green jackfruit, drained and rinsed well
- ½ cup water
- ¼ cup orange juice
- 1 tablespoon lime juice
- 1 teaspoon liquid smoke (optional)

Wet ingredients:

- 1 tablespoon tomato paste
- 2 tablespoons soy sauce
- 2 tablespoons avocado oil
- 2 tablespoons brown sugar
- 2 teaspoons cumin

- 1 teaspoon smoked paprika
- Himalayan salt and cayenne pepper to preference

Directions:

1. Preheat oven to 425°F. Line a baking sheet with parchment paper.
2. Place jackfruit onto a cutting board and chop off the hard center, core portions.
3. In a skillet, add olive oil and onion over medium heat. Cook for 4 minutes before adding in jackfruit and ½ cup of water.
4. Cover the skillet and simmer for 10 minutes.
5. In a bowl, mix all wet ingredients listed above.
6. After 10 minutes, remove the lid and use a fork to shred the jackfruit. Add the wet ingredients into the jackfruit and stir. Allow the jackfruit to simmer for 5 minutes, stirring occasionally.
7. Add in orange juice, lime juice, and liquid smoke. Simmer for an additional 10 minutes.
8. Spread the jackfruit mixture onto the baking sheet and bake for 20 minutes or until the jackfruit is crispy. Some spots may even blacken slightly.
9. Remove the jackfruit from oven and serve.

Note: The jackfruit should be served over a salad or used in tacos. Additional toppings like black beans, avocados, lettuce, and tomato should be served with the carnitas to add more nutrition and protein.

Lunch Recipe: Three

Chicken Salad

Nutritional Information Per Serving: 420 calories, 20 grams fat, 18 grams protein, 14 grams fiber, 52 grams carbs

Time: 15 minutes prep, 15 minutes total

Serving Size: 2 servings

Ingredients:

- 15 ounces (1 can) chickpeas, drained and rinsed
- ½ cup raw almonds, slivered
- 2 celery stalks, diced
- ½ cup grapes, halved
- ¼ cup dried cranberries
- ½ cup vegan mayo
- ½ lemon, juiced
- sea salt and black pepper to preference

Directions:

1. Add chickpeas and almonds to a food processor and pulse a few times. Do not over process, as the mixture should remain chunky.

2. Add the chickpeas and almond mixture to a large bowl. Add in all other ingredients and stir until everything is evenly combined.

3. Refrigerate until consumed. Serve alone, with crackers, over a salad, or as a sandwich with other desired toppings.

Lunch Recipe: Four

Thai Noodles

Nutritional Information Per Serving: 483 calories, 17 grams fat, 16 grams protein, 9 grams fiber, 70 grams carbs

Time: 15 minutes prep, 20 minutes total

Serving Size: 4 servings

Ingredients:

For the sauce:
- ½ cup peanut butter, natural
- ½ cup water
- ¼ cup coconut aminos
- 2 teaspoons garlic, minced
- 1 small lime, juiced
- 3 tablespoons maple syrup
- 1 teaspoon Sriracha

For the dish:
- 7 ounces stir fry noodles (substitute brown rice noodles if necessary)
- 2 cups cabbage
- 2 carrots, peeled and chopped

- 1 bell pepper, sliced
- 2 green onion, roughly chopped
- ¼ cup cilantro
- ¼ cup peanuts, roughly chopped

Directions:

1. Prepare the sauce by whisking together all sauce ingredients until a smooth consistency appears. Set the sauce aside.
2. Cook the noodles using the instructions on the packaging.
3. Add cabbage, carrots, red pepper, and onions to a pot. Add a dab of water to prevent burning and cook over medium heat for 5 minutes or until vegetables are soft. Stir frequently to prevent burning.
4. Combine sauce and vegetables to the pot containing the noodles. Stir well and let the pasta rest for 5 minutes. Serve warm or cold.

Lunch Recipe: Five

Broccoli Cheese Soup

Nutritional Information Per Serving: 245 calories, 9 grams fat, 11 grams protein, 7 grams fiber, 35 grams carbs

Time: 5 minutes prep, 30 minutes total

Serving Size: 4 servings

Ingredients:

- 2 tablespoons olive oil
- 1 small onion, roughly chopped
- 4 cups broccoli florets
- 2 teaspoons garlic, minced
- 1 medium potato, peeled and cubed
- 3 medium carrots, peeled and chopped
- ½ cup cashews, raw
- 4 cups vegetable broth
- ½ cup nutritional yeast
- 1 teaspoon smoked paprika
- 1 to 2 cups water
- sea salt and black pepper to preference

Directions:

1. Add onion, garlic, and olive oil to a large soup pot. Turn the heat to medium and sauté for 3 minutes.
2. Add the potato, carrots, cashews, vegetable broth, nutritional yeast, smoked paprika, salt, and pepper. Bring the content to a boil before reducing to low heat.
3. Simmer for 15 minutes, stirring occasionally.
4. Transfer the soup to a blender and blend until smooth. Return the soup to the pot when finished. Work in batches if needed.
5. Add in broccoli and one cup of water to the soup to reach a smooth consistency.
6. Bring to a boil, then allow the soup to simmer for 15 minutes. Serve warm.

Lunch Recipe: Six

Chickpea Tuna Salad

Nutritional Information Per Serving: 281 calories, 8 grams fat, 13 grams protein, 11 grams fiber, 40 grams carbs

Time: 10 minutes prep, 30 minutes total

Serving Size: 6 servings

Ingredients:

- 15 ounces (2 cans) chickpeas, drained and rinsed
- 2 medium dill pickles, chopped
- 1 or 2 celery stalks, chopped
- 4 tablespoons vegan mayo
- 1 tablespoon soy sauce
- sea salt and black pepper to preference

Directions:

1. Place the chickpeas into a small bowl and mash using a fork. The consistency should remain thick, with a few beans being left whole.
2. Add the remaining ingredients and mix until well combined.

3. Cover and refrigerate for 20 minutes to let the flavors come together.

4. Serve over salad, with crackers, as a wrap, or as a sandwich with additional toppings.

Lunch Recipe: Seven

Meal-Prep Protein Bowls

Nutritional Information Per Serving: 557 calories, 19 grams fat, 19 grams protein, 11 grams fiber, 80 grams carbs

Time: 15 minutes prep, 55 minutes total

Serving Size: 5 servings

Ingredients:

For the bowl:
- 1½ cup brown rice, uncooked
- 2 medium sweet potatoes
- 5 ounces (5 small handfuls per bowl) kale, chopped
- 15 ounces (1 can) black beans, drained and rinsed
- Himalayan salt and black pepper to preference

For the sauce:
- 1½ cups cashews, raw
- 1 cup water
- 1 teaspoon minced garlic
- hot sauce to preference (optional)

Directions:

1. Preheat the oven to 400°F. Line a baking sheet with parchment paper and spray with non-stick spray.
2. Place the rice into a medium pot. Add 3 cups of water and bring the rice to a boil. Reduce to low heat and simmer for 40 minutes.
3. Wash and chop the sweet potatoes into bite-sized cubes. Place the sweet potatoes onto the baking sheet. Sprinkle salt, pepper, and other desired spices over the potatoes. Bake for 30 minutes or until crispy. Remove and set aside when finished.
4. Set the cashews into a small bowl and pour boiling hot water over the top. Allow them to soak for at least 10 minutes.
5. Add the cashews to a blender along with 1 cup of water, garlic, hot sauce, salt, and pepper. Blend until a smooth sauce forms.
6. When all the ingredients are finished, gather 5 glass containers (or plates if consuming right away) to prep the bowls.
7. Start by layering the rice, beans, sweet potatoes, and kale. Evenly pour the sauce over each bowl. Store in the refrigerator until they are ready to be consumed.

Lunch Recipe: Eight

Mediterranean Tabbouleh Salad

Nutritional Information Per Serving: 412 calories, 24 grams fat, 10 grams protein, 6 grams fiber, 44 grams carbs

Time: 20 minutes prep, 55 minutes total

Serving Size: 4 servings

Ingredients:

For the salad:
- 1 cup quinoa
- 2 cups water
- 1½ cup chickpeas, drained and rinsed
- 2 cups cherry tomatoes, halved
- 2 cups cucumber, in small cubes
- ¾ cups fresh parsley, finely chopped
- ⅔ cups scallions, chopped
- 2 tablespoons mint, finely chopped
- sea salt and black pepper to preference

For the sauce:
- ⅓ cup olive oil, extra virgin
- 1½ lemons, juiced

- 1 or 2 teaspoons garlic, minced

Directions:

1. Cook the quinoa using the directions on the packaging. Afterwards, remove as much water as possible and place in the refrigerator until cool.
2. After preparing and chopping the vegetables, add the chickpeas, tomatoes, cucumbers, parsley, onion, mint, and spices to a large bowl.
3. In a canning jar or glass bottle, add all sauce ingredients and shake vigorously.
4. Pour the sauce over the vegetables and refrigerate. Serve chilled.

Lunch Recipe: Nine

Caesar Salad

Nutritional Information Per Serving: 429 calories, 26 grams fat, 17 grams protein, 9 grams fiber, 37 grams carbs

Time: 20 minutes prep, 55 minutes total

Serving Size: 6 servings

Ingredients:

For the croutons:
- 3 cups chickpeas, drained and rinsed
- 1 tablespoon avocado oil
- ¾ teaspoon onion powder
- ¾ teaspoon smoked paprika

For the dressing:
- 1¼ cups cashews, raw
- 1 cup water
- 2 teaspoons garlic, minced
- 1 medium lemon, juiced
- sea salt and black pepper to preference

For the cheese:

- 1 cup cashews, raw
- ¼ cup nutritional yeast
- ½ teaspoon garlic powder

For the salad:
- 3 medium heads of romaine lettuce, washed and chopped
- any other desired toppings (tomato, avocado, olives, etc.)

Directions:

1. Preheat the oven to 400°F. Line a baking sheet with parchment paper. Coat the parchment paper with a dab of oil or non-stick spray.
2. Place the chickpeas in a bowl with all other crouton ingredients. Toss to evenly coat before placing them on the baking sheet. Bake for 20 minutes.
3. Remove chickpeas from the oven and stir them around. Return them to the oven for an additional 20 minutes. They should be flaky and crispy. Set aside when finished.
4. While the chickpeas are cooking, prepare the dressing by pouring boiling hot water over the cashews. Allow the cashew to soak for 5 to 10 minutes.
5. Drain the cashews. Place the cashews and all other dressing ingredients into a high-speed

blender. Blend until a smooth consistency is achieved.

6. To prepare the cheese, place all cheese ingredients into a food processor or high-speed blender. Pulse until a crumbly texture appears. Store in the refrigerator until ready to be consumed.

7. When all of the elements are finished, assemble the salad by placing lettuce, dressing, croutons, and cheese into a bowl. Serve with other toppings if desired.

Lunch Recipe: Ten

Spicy Lentil Soup

Nutritional Information Per Serving: 236 calories, 4 grams fat, 13 grams protein, 16 grams fiber, 38 grams carbs

Time: 15 minutes prep, 45 minutes total

Serving Size: 8 servings

Ingredients:

- 2 tablespoon olive oil
- 1 medium onion, chopped
- 3 cloved garlic, minced
- 2 medium carrots, peeled and diced
- 2 celery stalks, chopped finely
- 14 ounces canned crushed tomatoes
- 2 cups lentils (green or brown)
- 7 cups vegetable broth
- ½ teaspoon ground cumin
- ½ teaspoon ground cumin
- 2 teaspoons smoked paprika
- 1 tablespoon cayenne pepper flakes (optional)
- 3 cups baby spinach
- 1 medium lemon, juiced
- Himalayan salt and pepper to preference

1. In a large soup pot, add olive oil, onions, garlic, carrots, and celery. Cook over medium heat and stir frequently for 5 minutes.
2. Add in tomatoes, lentils. vegetable broth, and spices. Mix well.
3. Bring the soup to a boil before reducing to low heat. Simmer for 30 minutes, stirring occasionally.
4. Stir in spinach and lemon juice. After 30 seconds, turn off the heat. Add in any additional spices, salt, or pepper.
5. Serve warm.

Lunch Recipe: Eleven

Pesto Sandwich

Nutritional Information Per Serving: 440 calories, 24 grams fat, 16 grams protein, 14 grams fiber, 49 grams carbs

Time: 10 minutes prep, 10 minutes total

Serving Size: 1 serving

Ingredients:

For the pesto:
- ¼ cup raw cashews
- ½ teaspoon garlic, minced
- ½ cup fresh basil
- 1 tablespoons nutritional yeast
- ½ tablespoon lemon juice
- 2 tablespoons water
- sea salt and pepper to preference

For the sandwich:
- 2 slices Ezekiel bread (whole grain, seeded bread)
- ½ tomato, sliced
- handful of lettuce

- ¼ whole cucumber, thinly sliced
- ½ avocado, mashed

Directions:

1. Add all pesto ingredients to a blender and blend until a smooth consistency is reached.
2. Assemble the sandwich by toasting the bread and chopping the toppings.
3. Place all ingredients onto the toast to form a sandwich.

Lunch Recipe: Twelve

Creamy Bacon Pasta Salad

Nutritional Information Per Serving: 440 calories, 10 grams fat, 20 grams protein, 4 grams fiber, 68 grams carbs

Time: 10 minutes prep, 30 minutes total

Serving Size: 6 servings

Ingredients:

For the pasta:
- 16 ounces rotini pasta
- 1 large tomato, diced
- 4 ounces black olives
- 1 cup carrots, shredded

For the dressing:
- 1½ cups cashews, raw
- ¾ cup water
- 2 tablespoons apple cider vinegar
- 1 lemon, juiced
- 1 teaspoon garlic powder
- 2 teaspoon onion powder
- 3 teaspoons dried dill

For the bacon:
- 8 ounces (1 package) tempeh
- ¼ cup soy sauce
- ¼ cup apple cider vinegar
- 1 tablespoon maple syrup
- ¼ teaspoon ground cumin
- 2 teaspoons liquid smoke

Directions:

1. To marinate the tempeh, add soy sauce, apple cider vinegar, maple syrup, cumin, and liquid smoke to a medium bowl. Using your hands, crumble in the tempeh. Stir, cover, and place in refrigerator for 20 minutes.
2. Prepare the dressing by covering the cashews with boiling hot water. Allow them to soak for 10 minutes. Drain and transfer to a blender when finished.
3. Add all other dressing ingredients to the blender, excluding the dill. Blend until smooth.
4. Stir in the dill using a spoon, or lightly pulse. Refrigerate until the other elements are done.
5. Prepare the pasta using the directions on the packaging. When finished, strain as much water as possible from the pasta.
6. Remove the tempeh from the refrigerator, drain, and pour into a small skillet. Add a dab of

oil to prevent burning or use a small amount of the marinade.

7. Turn the stove to medium heat and sauté the tempeh for 10 minutes. Stir frequently.

8. In a large bowl, combine all elements. Refrigerate and serve chilled.

Lunch Recipe: Thirteen

Quesadillas

Nutritional Information Per Serving: 403 calories, 24 grams fat, 16 grams protein, 5 grams fiber, 38 grams carbs

Time: 15 minutes prep, 30 minutes total

Serving Size: 4 servings

Ingredients:

For the cheese:
- 1 ½ cup cashews, raw
- ¼ cup nutritional yeast
- ¼ teaspoon garlic powder
- ½ teaspoon ground cumin
- ½ teaspoon chilli powder
- 6 tablespoons salsa

For the fillings:
- 15 ounces (1 can) black beans, drained and rinsed
- 1 small zucchini, finely chopped
- 2 small tomatoes, finely chopped
- handful of mushrooms, sliced

- 8 tortillas

Directions:

1. To make the cheese sauce, add the cashews to a food processor and blend for 4 minutes. A thick paste should begin to form.
2. Add in remaining cheese ingredients to the food processor and mix until well combined. Use a drop of water to reach desired consistency.
3. Heat a medium-sized, non-stick skillet over medium heat.
4. **Take a tortilla and spread ⅓ cup of cheese along with the black beans and vegetables. Cover the tortilla by placing an additional tortilla on top of the fillings.**
5. Place the tortilla in the pan and cook both sides until golden brown and flaky. This should take about 2 to 3 minutes on each side.
6. Serve warm with additional toppings or sauces if desired.

Lunch Recipe: Fourteen

Veggie Burgers

Nutritional Information Per Serving: 130 calories, 5 grams fat, 4 grams protein, 5 grams fiber, 18 grams carbs

Time: 30 minutes prep, 1 hour total

Serving Size: 8 servings

Ingredients:

- 2 cups chopped butternut squash
- 2 teaspoons garlic, minced
- 1 small shallot
- 15 ounces (1 can) white beans, drained and rinsed
- 3 chipotles in adobo sauce
- 2 flax eggs (2 tablespoons of ground flaxseed, 6 tablespoons water)
- 1 cup quinoa
- ⅔ cup rolled oats
- ⅓ cup flaxseed meal
- 2 teaspoons smoked paprika
- sea salt and black pepper to preference

Directions:

1. Prepare the flax egg by mixing the ingredients together. Place in the refrigerator for 15 minutes.
2. Line a baking sheet with parchment paper.
3. Add butternut squash, shallots, and garlic to a food processor. Pulse a few times before adding in all remaining ingredients.
4. Split the dough into 8 parts and form patties. Place on baking sheet or plate and refrigerate for 30 minutes.
5. Preheat oven to 375°F.
6. Bake the burgers for 20 minutes. Flip the patties and return the patties to the oven for an additional 20 minutes. Total bake time is 40 minutes.
7. Remove the patties and allow cooling. Serve warm on a bun, over a salad, or in a wrap with additional toppings.

Lunch Recipe: Fifteen

Buffalo Wraps

Nutritional Information Per Serving: 330 calories, 8 grams fat, 12 grams protein, 7 grams fiber, 50 grams carbs

Time: 10 minutes prep, 50 minutes total

Serving Size: 4 servings

Ingredients:

For the cauliflower:
- 4 cups cauliflower, in florets
- ¾ cup almond flour
- 2/4 cup almond milk, unsweetened
- ½ cup buffalo sauce
- 1 teaspoon garlic powder
- Himalayan salt and black pepper to preference

For the sauce:
- 1 package tofu, soft
- 3 tablespoons lemon juice
- 1 tablespoon apple cider vinegar
- 2 teaspoons onion powder
- handful of parsley, roughly chopped

For the wraps:
- 4 handfuls of lettuce (1 handful for each wrap)
- ½ cucumber, thinly sliced
- 2 carrot stalks, grated
- 2 avocados, mashed
- 4 large tortillas

Directions:

1. Preheat the oven to 425°F. Line a baking sheet with parchment paper.
2. In a large bowl, mix almond flour, almond milk, garlic powder, salt, and pepper. Let the batter rest for 5 minutes. The batter should be smooth and slightly runny.
3. Combine the cauliflower florets with the batter. Coat all florets evenly before pouring onto the baking sheet.
4. Bake the cauliflower for 25 minutes, then remove from oven.
5. Coat the florets with the buffalo sauce. Use the same bowl as before to save time later.
6. Return the florets to the oven for an additional 15 minutes or until brown.
7. While the cauliflower cooks, place all sauce ingredients in a blender and pulse until well combined.

8. Once all of the elements are finished, assemble
    the wraps by evenly distributing the ingredients
    among the wraps.

Lunch Recipe: Sixteen

Asian Slaw

Nutritional Information Per Serving: 484 calories, 30 grams fat, 10 grams protein, 8 grams fiber, 47 grams carbs

Time: 20 minutes prep, 20 minutes total

Serving Size: 4 servings

Ingredients:

For the salad:
- ⅓ cup cashews, chopped
- 1 tablespoon sesame seeds
- 6 cups cabbage, shredded
- 1 cup quinoa, cooked
- 1 cup carrots, shredded
- ¼ cup cilantro, roughly chopped
- 2 green onions, chopped

For the dressing:
- ½ cup apple cider vinegar
- ½ cup water
- 1 teaspoon ginger, grated
- 1 teaspoon garlic, minced

- 1 tablespoon maple syrup
- 2 tablespoons olive oil, extra virgin

Directions:

1. Preheat the oven to 350°F. Line a baking sheet with parchment paper.
2. Place the cashews and sesame seeds on the baking sheet and roast for 5 minutes. The nuts and seeds should be golden brown. Set aside when finished and allow cooling.
3. Place all dressing ingredients in a blender or canning jar. Mix until well combined and creamy.
4. In a large bowl, chop and combine all salad ingredients. Toss with dressing and serve chilled.

Lunch Recipe: Seventeen

Cream of Mushroom Soup

Nutritional Information Per Serving: 250 calories, 17 grams fat, 7 grams protein, 3 grams fiber, 15 grams carbs

Time: 10 minutes prep, 25 minutes total

Serving Size: 3 servings

Ingredients:

- 3 tablespoons olive oil, extra virgin
- 3 cups mushrooms, sliced
- 1 small onion, finely chopped
- 2 teaspoons garlic, minced
- ½ cup chickpea flour (substitute all-purpose if necessary)
- 2 cups almond milk, unsweetened
- 1 tablespoon dry white wine (optional)
- ¼ teaspoon nutmeg
- Himalayan salt and black pepper to preference

Directions:

1. Add olive oil to a soup pot over medium heat. Warm for a minute before adding in mushrooms and onion. Sauté for 4 minutes until the vegetables are tender.
2. Add the chickpea flour to the vegetables and stir. This roux will help thicken the soup.
3. Add white wine, almond milk, and spices to the pot. Stir frequently until everything is well combined.
4. Bring the soup to a boil, then reduce to low heat. Allow the soup to simmer for 10 minutes. Stir occasionally.
5. Remove from heat and serve warm.

Lunch Recipe: Eighteen

Italian Pasta Salad

Nutritional Information Per Serving: 240 calories, 15 grams fat, 4 grams protein, 2 grams fiber, 23 grams carbs

Time: 10 minutes prep, 25 minutes total

Serving Size: 6 servings

Ingredients:

For the salad:
- 1½ cups noodles of choice
- ½ cup packed artichoke hearts, chopped
- ¼ cup capers, chopped
- ¼ cup kalamata olives
- 1 tablespoon oregano

For the dressing:
- ⅓ cup olive oil, extra virgin
- 2 tablespoons apple cider vinegar
- 1 tablespoon lemon juice
- 2 teaspoons dijon mustard
- 1 teaspoon garlic, minced
- sea salt and black pepper to preference

Directions:

1. Prepare the noodles using the instructions on the packaging. When the noodles are soft, drain and place in the refrigerator for cooling.
2. Place all dressing ingredients into a canning jar and shake vigorously. A blender can also be used.
3. Combine all ingredients with the dressing in a large bowl. Mix well and serve chilled.

Lunch Recipe: Nineteen

Stir Fry with Bean Sauce

Nutritional Information Per Serving: 155 calories, 10 grams fat, 5 grams protein, 7 grams fiber, 20 grams carbs

Time: 15 minutes prep, 30 minutes total

Serving Size: 4 servings

Ingredients:

For the sauce:
- ½ cup black beans, drained and rinsed
- 1 tablespoon dry sherry
- 2 tablespoons vegetable broth
- 1 tablespoon soy sauce
- 1 tablespoon maple syrup
- 1 teaspoon garlic, minced

For the vegetables:
- 2 tablespoons coconut oil, melted
- 1 large eggplant, chopped
- 1 medium onion, chopped
- 1 teaspoon ginger
- 2 small zucchinis, chopped

- ½ red bell pepper, sliced
- ½ cup cabbage, thinly chopped (optional)

Directions:

1. To prepare the sauce, add all ingredients to a high-speed blender. Blend until smooth. Transfer the sauce into a small saucepan.
2. Heat the sauce over low heat for 15 minutes. Cover and remove from heat when finished.
3. In a mixing bowl, add the chopped eggplant. Pour in 1 tablespoon coconut oil and toss to evenly coat.
4. Add the eggplant to a large skillet and turn the stove to medium heat. Sauté for 5 minutes then empty the skillet, and set the eggplant aside.
5. Heat 1 tablespoon of coconut oil in the same skillet used before over medium heat.
6. Add onions, ginger, and garlic. Sauté for 2 minutes.
7. Add in zucchini and bell pepper. Sauté for 3 minutes. Stir frequently.
8. Add cabbage and sauté for 3 minutes.
9. Add the eggplant and sauce into the skillet containing the vegetables and stir to incorporate everything.
10. Serve warm alone, or serve over rice or asian noodles.

Lunch Recipe: Twenty

Spaghetti Squash Mac

Nutritional Information Per Serving: 350 calories, 6 grams fat, 26 grams protein, 18 grams fiber, 55 grams carbs

Time: 15 minutes prep, 1 hour and 15 minutes total

Serving Size: 2 servings

Ingredients:

- 1 large spaghetti squash
- 2 cups broccoli, in florets
- 1½ cups oat milk
- 4 tablespoons Dijon mustard
- 2 tablespoons soy sauce
- ¾ cup nutritional yeast
- 2 tablespoons flour
- 2 teaspoons onion powder
- sea salt and black pepper to preference

Directions:

1. Preheat oven to 400°F. Line a baking sheet with aluminum foil.

2. Spice the squash in half. Place on baking sheet and roast in the oven for 1 hour.
3. Place broccoli florets in a microwave-safe bowl. Add 2 tablespoons of water, cover, and microwave on high for 4 minutes.
4. Combine all other ingredients (everything excluding broccoli and squash) in a blender. Pulse until smooth.
5. When the squash is done baking, carefully remove the seeds from the squash, then take a fork and scrape out the squash. The squash should resemble noodles.
6. Combine all elements in a large bowl and serve warm.

Chapter 4:

Dinner

This section will take you through recipes for dinner. Dinner is an important meal for a bodybuilder, as many workouts take place in the evening. Even if you prefer to workout in the morning, dinner is a time to nourish the body before a night of recovery. Many of these recipes are great to bring to dinner parties. Many individuals are unaware of how tasty vegan foods can be, so spread the message!

Dinner Recipe: One

Enchiladas

Nutritional Information Per Serving: 375 calories, 15 grams fat, 16 grams protein, 13 grams fiber, 52 grams carbs

Time: 25 minutes prep, 50 minutes total

Serving Size: 6 servings

Ingredients:

For the sauce:
- 2 cups vegetable broth
- 3 tablespoons water
- 3 tablespoons all-purpose flour
- 3 tablespoons taco seasonings
- 2 tablespoons tomato paste
- 1 teaspoon apple cider vinegar
- sea salt and cayenne pepper to preference

For the meat:
- ½ medium cauliflower head, in large florets
- 5 medium-sized mushrooms, sliced
- ½ cup walnuts, raw
- 1 teaspoon smoked paprika

- 1 teaspoon garlic powder
- 2 tablespoons soy sauce

For the dish:
- 15 ounces (1 can) black beans, drained and rinsed
- 15 corn tortillas
- ¼ cup cilantro, chopped
- 1 cup raw cashews
- 1 tablespoon lemon juice
- 2 cups water
- ¼ cup nutritional yeast
- 2 teaspoons taco seasoning
- 2 teaspoons Sriracha or hot sauce

Directions:

For the dish:
1. To prepare the dish, place the cashews in a bowl and pour over boiling hot water to soak. Allow the cashews to soak for 15 minutes before draining.
2. Add the cashews, lemon juice, 2 cups of water, nutritional yeast, taco seasoning and Sriracha to a blender. Blend until smooth to create cheese sauce, then set aside.

For the sauce:

3. To prepare the sauce, add all dry sauce ingredients to a small bowl.

4. Add 3 tablespoons of water to a pot and turn to medium heat. After a minute, add all dry ingredients and whisk vigorously for 1 minute. Add in tomato paste, then broth.

5. Bring the sauce to a boil then turn to low heat. Simmer for 5 minutes. Stir frequently to avoid lumps and to create a smooth texture.

6. Remove from heat and add in the last ingredient, vinegar. Set aside when finished.

For the meat:

7. To prepare the meat, add cauliflower, mushrooms, and walnuts to a food processor. Pulse until medium-sized crumbles appear. Do not overproccess.

8. Add the crumbles to a pan over medium heat and pour in 2 tablespoons of vegetable broth.

9. Add in meat spices and soy sauce. Stir to make sure the elements are well incorporated.

10. Sauté for 15 minutes, stirring frequently to avoid burning.

11. Stir in black beans and turn the heat off.

To assemble:

12. Preheat oven to 375°F. Set aside a 9 x 13 inch casserole dish.

13. Start by spreading ½ cup of the sauce into the bottom of the dish.
14. Wrap 5 tortillas in a paper towel and microwave for 30 seconds to dampen.
15. Fill each tortilla with a scoop of meat and a scoop of the cheese sauce. Roll and place in the pan.
16. Repeat steps 14 and 15 until no tortillas remain. Pour the sauce over each tortilla at the end. Pour any leftover cheese sauce and meat over the top.
17. Bake for 25 minutes. Serve warm and top with cilantro or any other desired toppings.

Dinner Recipe: Two

Twice-Baked Potatoes

Nutritional Information Per Serving: 460 calories, 14 grams fat, 16 grams protein, 10 grams fiber, 74 grams carbs

Time: 30 minutes prep, 1 hour and 35 minutes total

Serving Size: 4 servings

Ingredients:

- 4 large potatoes
- 5 cups broccoli, in florets
- 2 cups vegan cheese shreds
- 2 cups butternut squash, cubed
- ½ cup cashews, raw
- 2 cups water
- 2 tablespoons cornstarch
- ½ cup nutritional yeast
- 1 tablespoon yellow mustard
- 1 teaspoon onion powder
- 2 tablespoons lemon juice
- sea salt and black pepper to preference

Directions:

1. Add cashews to a bowl and pour boiling hot water over them. Set aside.
2. Preheat oven to 350°F. Set aside 2 baking sheets.
3. Clean the potatoes to remove debris. Prick the potatoes using a fork and lightly coat with olive oil.
4. Place the cubed butternut squash onto a lined baking sheet. Bake for 20 to 25 minutes until the squash is soft.
5. Set potatoes onto the sheet and bake the potatoes for 1 hour and 15 minutes or until potatoes are soft. Allow the potatoes to cool for 15 minutes.
6. When the squash is finished, drain the cashews.
7. Add the cashews, squash, 2 cups of water, cornstarch, mustard, garlic powder, onion powder, lemon juice, salt and pepper to a blender. Blend until smooth to create the cheese sauce.
8. Steam the broccoli by placing the florets in a large saucepan. Add one inch of water and turn the heat to medium. Cook until tender or for about 8 minutes.
9. When potatoes are finished and cooled, slice them in half. Remove the potato contents and place them into a large bowl. The potatoes should retain their shape, so don't scoop out everything.

10. Add ¾ of the sauce to the bowl containing the potato contents. Mash until well incorporated.
11. Stir in the steamed broccoli.
12. Spoon the mixture evenly, back into the potatoes. Sprinkle vegan cheese shreds over the top.
13. Bake for 20 minutes.
14. Serve warm with additional cheese sauce drizzled over the top.

Dinner Recipe: Three

Red Thai Curry

Nutritional Information Per Serving: 208 calories, 14 grams fat, 5 grams protein, 3 grams fiber, 15 grams carbs

Time: 10 minutes prep, 30 minutes total

Serving Size: 6 servings

Ingredients:

- 1 small onion, chopped
- 2 teaspoons garlic, minced
- 1 tablespoon ginger, grated
- 1 red bell pepper, thinly sliced
- 2 medium carrots, peeled and sliced
- 2 cup cauliflower, florets
- 2½ tablespoons thai red curry paste
- 15 ounces (1 can) coconut milk, full fat
- ½ cup vegetable broth
- 2 cups baby spinach
- 1 medium tomatoes, diced
- 2 tablespoons soy sauce
- 1 small lime, juiced
- sea salt and black pepper to preference

Directions:

1. Prepare all vegetables and keep them nearby.
2. In a large skillet, add a few tablespoons of water over medium heat. Add in onion, garlic, and ginger. Sauté for 1 or 2 minutes.
3. Add in bell peppers, carrots, and cauliflower. Sauté for 5 minutes, stirring frequently to prevent burning. Use water as needed.
4. Add in curry paste, coconut milk, and vegetable broth. Mix well.
5. Bring the contents to a boil, then reduce to low heat. Cover and allow the vegetables to simmer for 10 minutes.
6. Add in tomatoes, spinach, soy sauce, and lime juice. Stir until well combined, then remove from heat.
7. Serve warm over rice, potatoes, noodles, or grain of choice.

Dinner Recipe: Four

Fettuccini

Nutritional Information Per Serving: 570 calories, 5 grams fat, 20 grams protein, 11 grams fiber, 70 grams carbs

Time: 10 minutes prep, 25 minutes total

Serving Size: 3 servings

Ingredients:

For the sauce:
- 2 tablespoons olive oil
- 3 teaspoons garlic, minced
- 6 cups cauliflower, florets
- ¾ cup cashews, raw
- 3 cups vegetable broth
- sea salt and black pepper to preference

For the pasta:
- 6 ounces fettuccine pasta
- 3 cups broccoli, in florets
- 1 tablespoon lemon juice (optional)
- sea salt and black pepper to preference

Directions:

1. Cook the pasta using the directions on the packaging. Drain and return the pasta to the pot when finished.
2. Steam the broccoli by placing the florets into a saucepan. Add 1 inch of water and cover. Simmer over low heat for 10 minutes or until the broccoli is tender. Stir occasionally.
3. To prepare the sauce, add garlic and olive oil to a medium saucepan. Simmer for 2 minutes over medium heat.
4. Add cauliflower, cashews, and vegetable broth. Stir and bring the contents to a boil. Reduce to medium-low heat and cook for 15 minutes.
5. Transfer to a blender and blend until smooth. Return the sauce to the pot containing the noodles.
6. Add in broccoli, salt, pepper, and other spices or vegetables. Drizzle lemon juice over the top. Serve warm.

Dinner Recipe: Five

Stuffed Shells

Nutritional Information Per Serving: 425 calories, 3 grams fat, 20 grams protein, 6 grams fiber, 52 grams carbs

Time: 10 minutes prep, 45 minutes total

Serving Size: 8 servings

Ingredients:

For the dish:
- 12 ounces (1 package) jumbo shells
- 3 cups marinara sauce, organic
- sea salt and black pepper to preference

For the ricotta:
- 2 cups cashews, raw
- 14 ounces (1 package) tofu, firm
- ½ cup nutritional yeast
- 1 large lemon, juiced
- ¼ cup vegetable broth
- 3 teaspoons oregano
- 1 teaspoon onion powder
- 1 teaspoon garlic powder

- 10 ounces (1 package) frozen spinach, thawed

Directions:

1. Preheat oven to 350°F.
2. Fill a large pot with water and bring to a boil. Add the shells and cook for 10 minutes or until done (refer to instructions on packaging). Drain and rinse the shells with cold water.
3. To make the ricotta, add the cashews to a food processor. Pulse until a fine and crumbly texture appears. Add all other ricotta ingredients, excluding the spinach. Blend until smooth, then pulse in the spinach.
4. In a large casserole dish, evenly spread 1 cup of marinara sauce onto the bottom of the dish.
5. Stuff the pasta by scooping 2 tablespoons of ricotta into the shell. Repeat and place each shell in the dish with the open part facing upwards.
6. When all the ricotta has been used, pour over the remaining marinara sauce.
7. Bake the shells for 25 minutes. Afterwards, allow 5 minutes of cooling and serve warm.

Dinner Recipe: Six

Fried Rice Scramble

Nutritional Information Per Serving: 550 calories, 12 grams fat, 26 grams protein, 12 grams fiber, 85 grams carbs

Time: 10 minutes prep, 40 minutes total

Serving Size: 3 servings

Ingredients:

For the tofu:
- 2 tablespoons water
- 16 ounces tofu, firm
- 1 teaspoon turmeric
- 2 tablespoons nutritional yeast
- 1 teaspoon onion powder
- sea salt and black pepper to preference

For the sauce:
- ⅓ cup soy sauce
- 6 tablespoons maple syrup, organic
- 2 teaspoons garlic, minced
- 3 teaspoons sesame oil (substitute melted coconut oil)

For the rice:
- 3 cups brown rice, cooked
- 1 cup green onions, roughly chopped
- 1 cup peas
- 1 cup carrots, diced
- 1 cup broccoli, small florets

Directions:

1. To prepare the tofu, heat 2 tablespoons of water over medium heat for 1 minute.
2. Crumble in the tofu using your hands. Cook for about 10 minutes or until the water from the tofu has evaporated. Stir frequently.
3. Add in all tofu ingredients and mix well to incorporate. Cook for an additional 3 minutes, then remove from heat.
4. To prepare the sauce, add all ingredients to a small bowl and whisk until smooth. A blender can also be used.
5. To prepare the rice, add carrots, broccoli, and ½ cup of water to a large skillet.
6. Simmer over medium heat for 5 minutes, stirring frequently.
7. Add the cooked rice, green onions, peas, scrambled tofu, and sauce. Simmer for an additional 10 minutes then serve.

Dinner Recipe: Seven

Pizza Crust

Nutritional Information Per Serving: 320 calories, 2 grams fat, 15 grams protein, 11 grams fiber, 65 grams carbs

Time: 10 minutes prep, 20 minutes total

Serving Size: 2 pizzas, 4 servings

Ingredients:

- 1 cup boiling hot water
- 2¼ teaspoon instant yeast
- 1 tablespoon sugar
- 2¾ cup whole wheat flour
- ¼ cup nutritional yeast
- 1 teaspoon salt

Directions:

1. Preheat oven to 425°F. Set aside pizza pans or a lightly greased baking sheet.
2. Add hot water, yeast, and sugar to a large bowl and whisk vigorously for 30 seconds. Leave the dough to rest for 5 minutes.

3. Add flour, nutritional yeast, and salt to the bowl containing the dough. Stir by hand or using a wooden spoon until mixture is well combined.
4. Transfer the dough onto a floured surface and knead by hand for 5 minutes. Form the dough into a ball.
5. Separate the dough into 2 equal parts.
6. Roll out the dough thin to fit pizza pans or baking sheet. Transfer the dough.
7. Add desired pizza sauce and toppings of choice.
8. Bake the pizza for 8 to 10 minutes. Remove the pizza from the oven and let cool.

Dinner Recipe: Eight

Buffalo Casserole

Nutritional Information Per Serving: 280 calories, 6 grams fat, 12 grams protein, 6 grams fiber, 46 grams carbs

Time: 10 minutes prep, 50 minutes total

Serving Size: 3 servings

Ingredients:

- 1 cup quinoa
- 3 cups cauliflower, in florets
- 1½ cup oat milk
- ½ cup vegan yogurt, unsweetened
- ½ cup buffalo sauce
- sea salt and black pepper to preference

Directions:

1. Preheat oven to 375°F. Gather a 9 x 9 inch baking dish.
2. Add the quinoa and cauliflower into the baking dish.
3. In a separate bowl, beat all wet ingredients until smooth.

4. Pour the wet ingredients into the baking dish, over the cauliflower. Stir to combine.

5. Bake for 45 minutes or until little to no liquid remains.

6. Serve warm with any other additional vegan toppings like chives, nutritional yeast, vegan cheese, or hot sauce.

Dinner Recipe: Nine

Sesame Garlic Zoodles

Nutritional Information Per Serving: 330 calories, 29 grams fat, 10 grams protein, 3 grams fiber, 13 grams carbs

Time: 10 minutes

Serving Size: 2 servings

Ingredients:

- 2 tablespoons tahini
- 2 tablespoons sesame oil
- 1 small lime, juiced
- 1 teaspoon garlic, minced
- 2 large zucchini
- ¼ cup pepitas, roasted/salted (for garnish)
- sesame seeds (for garnish)
- sea salt and black pepper to preference

Directions:

1. Use a spiralizer to create noodles using the zucchini. If you do not own a spiralizer, cut the zucchini into thin strips.

2. Add the zucchini into a skillet and add olive oil. Sauté on low heat for 3 to 5 minutes until the zucchini is soft. Do not overcook, as the zucchini will become mushy. Stir frequently. Remove from heat when finished.
3. Add all other ingredients to a canning jar and shake vigorously. A blender or whisk can also achieve the same effect.
4. Pour the sauce into the zucchini noodles and stir.
5. Serve warm and sprinkle over sesame seeds and pepitas to garnish.

Dinner Recipe: Ten

Stroganoff

Nutritional Information Per Serving: 385 calories, 16 grams fat, 21 grams protein, 10 grams fiber, 45 grams carbs

Time: 10 minutes prep, 30 minutes total

Serving Size: 4 servings

Ingredients:

- 8 ounces pasta
- 2 tablespoons olive oil
- ½ cup shallots, diced
- 2 teaspoons garlic, minced
- 1 lb mushrooms
- 1 tablespoon thyme, fresh
- 3 tablespoons flour
- 2½ cups vegetable broth
- ⅓ cup nutritional yeast
- ⅓ cup almond milk
- 2 teaspoons lemon juice
- sea salt and black pepper to preference

Directions:

1. To prepare the sauce, add 1 tablespoon of olive oil and shallots to a large skillet. Sauté over medium heat for 2 minutes.
2. Add remaining oil, garlic, mushrooms, and thyme. Sauté for an additional 5 minutes.
3. Add salt, pepper, and flour. Mix to well incoorperate.
4. Stir in vegetable broth. Turn the heat to low and allow everything to simmer for 5 minutes. Stir occasionally. The sauce should start to thicken.
5. Prepare the noodles by using the instructions on the packaging. When finished, drain and set aside.
6. Add nutritional yeast, almond milk, and lemon juice to the skillet containing the sauce.
7. Add in pasta and mix well.
8. Let the pasta simmer in the sauce for one minute, then remove from heat and serve.

Dinner Recipe: Eleven

Anti-Inflammatory Carrot Soup

Nutritional Information Per Serving: 210 calories, 11 grams fat, 2 grams protein, 5 grams fiber, 26 grams carbs

Time: 10 minutes prep, 50 minutes total

Serving Size: 4 servings

Ingredients:

- 1 tablespoon olive oil
- 1 leek, cleaned and sliced
- 4 cups celery, chopped
- 1 teaspoon fennel
- 4 cups carrots, chopped
- 3 teaspoons garlic, minced
- 1 tablespoon ginger, grated
- 1 tablespoon turmeric powder
- 3 cups vegetable broth
- 15 ounces canned coconut milk, light
- sea salt and black pepper to preference

Directions:

1. In a large saucepan, add olive oil, celery, leeks, and carrots. Sauté for 5 minutes over medium-low heat.
2. Add garlic, ginger, turmeric, fennel, salt, and pepper. Sauté for 3 minutes, stirring frequently. Add broth and coconut milk.
3. Bring the contents to a boil, then reduce, cover, and simmer over low heat for 20 minutes.
4. When the vegetables are soft, add the soup to a blender. Work in batches if necessary. Blend until smooth and return to pot.
5. Add any additional seasonings if desired and serve warm with your favorite bread.

Dinner Recipe: Twelve

Fresh Tostadas

Nutritional Information Per Serving: 280 calories, 14 grams of fat, 8 grams protein, 8 grams of fiber, 38 grams carbs

Time: 10 minutes prep, 10 minutes total

Serving Size: 3 servings

Ingredients:

- 1½ cups cucumber, chopped
- 1 cup cherry tomatoes, halved
- ½ cup black olives
- ¼ cup red onion, roughly chopped (optional)
- ¼ cup cilantro, roughly chopped
- 1 tablespoon olive oil
- ½ lemon, juiced
- 6 corn tortillas
- ½ cup hummus of choice
- ⅓ cup tahini
- sea salt and black pepper to preference

Directions:

1. In a medium-sized mixing bowl, add all vegetables and herbs. Toss until well incorporated.
2. Add olive oil, lemon juice, salt, and pepper to the bowl containing the vegetables. Stir or shake.
3. Prepare the tostadas by tossing the tortilla. This can be done over medium heat on the stovetop. Oil is not necessary, but be sure to constantly flip the tortillas to prevent burning.
4. When the tortillas are crispy, add a layer of hummus before topping with the vegetable salad.
5. Add the tahini to a small bowl and add water as needed to reach the desired consistency.
6. Drizzle the tahini evenly over the top of the tostadas.
7. Serve and enjoy.

Dinner Recipe: Thirteen

Chick'n Nuggets

Nutritional Information Per Serving: 410 calories, 17 grams fat, 20 grams protein, 16 grams fiber, 68 grams carbs

Time: 10 minutes prep, 30 minutes total

Serving Size: 2 servings

Ingredients:

- ½ cup panko
- ½ cup rolled oats
- 15 ounces (1 can) garbanzo beans
- 1 teaspoon onion powder
- 1 teaspoon salt
- black pepper to preference

Directions:

1. Preheat oven to 375°F. Set aside a baking sheet.
2. Pour panko onto the baking sheet and bake for 5 minutes. This will toast the panko and it should look golden brown afterwards. Transfer to a bowl when finished.

3. In a food processor, process the oats until a thin flour appears. Add the oat flour to a clean, separate bowl and set aside.
4. Drain the chickpeas over a bowl, and save ¼ cup of the liquid. Discard the rest.
5. Add the chickpeas to the food processor, along with salt and onion powder. Pulse until crumbly. Leave the mixture in the processor.
6. Whisk the chickpea liquid in a small bowl until foamy.
7. Add the foamy liquid and ½ the oat flour to the food processor. Pulse until the contents form a ball, adding oat flour as necessary.
8. Divide the dough into 12 equal parts and shape into a nugget.
9. Coat each nugget in the panko mixture before transferring onto a parchment paper, lined baking sheet.
10. Bake the nuggets for 15 to 20 minutes. Serve warm alongside any vegan dipping sauce.

Dinner Recipe: Fourteen

Barbecue Salad

Nutritional Information Per Serving: 455 calories, 25 grams fat, 6 grams protein, 6 grams fiber, 55 grams carbs

Time: 10 minutes prep, 15 minutes total

Serving Size: 2 servings

Ingredients:

- 2 cups chickpeas, drained and rinsed
- ½ cup barbecue sauce of choice
- 6 cups romaine lettuce, washed and chopped
- 1 cup cherry tomatoes, halved
- 1 cup cucumber, sliced
- 1 cup corn
- ¼ cup red onion, sliced
- 6 tablespoons dressing (try *Lunch Recipe: 12* or substitute your own)
- sea salt and black pepper to preference

Directions:

1. Add chickpeas and barbecue sauce to a saucepan. Toss to incorporate the sauce and

simmer on medium heat for 10 minutes. Stir occasionally to prevent burning. The sauce should become sticky. Remove from heat when finished.

2. Assemble the salads by evenly distributing the lettuce among 2 bowls. Separate and add the vegetables to each bowl before pouring over the chickpeas.

3. Complete the salad by pouring over your dressing of choice or extra barbecue sauce.

Dinner Recipe: Fifteen

Spaghetti Meatballs

Nutritional Information Per Serving: 374 calories, 4 grams fat, 19 grams protein, 13 grams fiber, 67 grams carbs

Time: 10 minutes prep, 35 minutes total

Serving Size: 2 servings

Ingredients:

- 15 ounces (1 can) chickpeas, drained and rinsed
- 3 garlic cloves
- ½ cup rolled oats
- 2 teaspoon oregano
- 2 tablespoons nutritional yeast
- ½ lemon, juiced
- 1 cup zucchini, shredded
- sea salt and black pepper to preference

Directions:

1. Preheat the oven to 375°F and line a baking sheet with parchment paper.

2. In a blender or food processor, add chickpeas, garlic, and rolled oats. Pulse for 10 seconds, then transfer the contents into a large bowl.

3. Add herbs, salt, nutritional yeast, lemon juice, and shredded zucchini to the bowl containing the chickpea mixture. Stir to incorporate. The mixture should be quite dry. Add extra nutritional yeast if necessary to soak up any moisture.

4. Separate the dough into 12 equal parts and roll into round meatballs. Set the meatballs onto the baking sheet.

5. Bake for 25 minutes or until golden brown.

6. Serve warm over pasta or in a sandwich with your favorite vegan marinara.

Dinner Recipe: Sixteen

Slow Cooker Sloppy Joe Bowls

Nutritional Information Per Serving: 355 calories, 3 grams fat, 16 grams protein, 13 grams fiber, 70 grams carbs

Time: 10 minutes prep, 4 hours and 10 minutes total

Serving Size: 4 servings

Ingredients:

- 1¼ cups green lentils, rinsed and drained
- 1 onion, diced
- 1 red pepper, diced
- 1 carrot, diced
- 2 teaspoons garlic, minced
- 1 tablespoon chili powder
- 1 teaspoon cumin
- 1 teaspoon onion powder
- 15 ounces (1 can) marinara
- 15 ounces (1 can) diced tomatoes
- 1½ cup water
- 2 tablespoons ketchup
- 1 teaspoon yellow mustard
- 1 spaghetti squash

- sea salt, cayenne, and black pepper to preference

Directions:

1. Add all ingredients except spaghetti squash to a slow cooker. Stir to incorporate.
2. Cut the squash in half and scoop out the seeds.
3. Place the squash face down on top of the contents in the slow cooker.
4. Cover and cook on high for 4 hours or until the squash and lentils are soft. Add water as necessary, but keep a thick consistency.
5. Remove the squash and shred using a fork.
6. Equally divide the squash among serving bowls before topping with the sloppy joe mixture. Serve warm.

Dinner Recipe: Seventeen

Stuffed Peppers

Nutritional Information Per Serving: 310 calories, 3 grams fat, 14 grams protein, 11 grams fiber, 60 grams carbs

Time: 10 minutes prep, 1 hour and 15 minutes total

Serving Size: 4 servings

Ingredients:

- 15 ounces (1 can) black beans, drained and rinsed
- 1 cup corn, drained
- 1 cup rice
- 2 cups vegetable stock
- 4 large bell peppers, seeded and halved
- ½ cup salsa
- 1 tablespoon nutritional yeast
- 1 tablespoon coconut oil, melted
- 1½ tablespoons taco seasoning
- sea salt and black pepper to preference

Directions:

1. Preheat oven to 375°F. Lightly grease a 9 x 13 inch baking dish.
2. Add vegetable stock and rice to a saucepan. Bring to a boil, then reduce to low heat. Cover and simmer for 20 minutes or until no liquid remains. Set aside when finished.
3. Brush the outside of the peppers using the melted coconut oil.
4. When the rice is finished, add to a large bowl. Mix in remaining ingredients and spices.
5. Distribute the rice mixture evenly among the peppers. Place the peppers into the baking dish, facing up, and cover with tinfoil.
6. Bake for 30 minutes. Then, remove the foil and increase heat to 400°F.
7. Bake for an additional 20 minutes until the peppers are golden brown in color.
8. Serve warm with any other desired toppings like salsa, avocado, cilantro, hot sauce, or vegan cheese.

Dinner Recipe: Eighteen

Vegan Ground Beef Recipe

Nutritional Information Per Serving (¼ lb): 360 calories, 4 grams fat, 26 grams protein, 25 grams fiber, 58 grams carbs

Time: 10 minutes prep, 20 minutes total

Serving Size: 6 servings

Ingredients:

- 2 cups brown lentils, rinsed
- 15 ounces (1 can) beets, drained
- 6 ounces mushrooms, quartered
- ½ onion, diced
- ½ cup nutritional yeast
- ⅓ cup coconut flour
- ¼ cup flaxseed meal
- 2 teaspoons onion powder
- 1 teaspoon smoked paprika
- sea salt and black pepper to preference

Directions:

1. Add the lentils to a saucepan. Cover with water by at least 1 inch. Bring to a boil, then reduce to

low heat. Simmer for 10 minutes, then drain and rinse with cool water.

2. Place lentils into a food processor. Pulse a few times only to keep a thick texture. Pour lentils into a bowl when finished.

3. Press the beets using paper towel and remove as water as possible. Then add to the food processor.

4. Add mushrooms and onions to the food processor and pulse until the texture is fine, but not a puree.

5. Add the mixture to the lentils and stir.

6. Add in all remaining ingredients.

7. Shape the meat into hamburgers.

8. Add a dab of oil in a non-stick skillet and cook each burger for 3 to 6 minutes, depending on the size of the burger. Be careful not to burn the patty.

9. Remove the burger and serve with a bun and your favorite hamburger toppings!

Dinner Recipe: Nineteen

Tofu Steak with Caramelized Gravy

Nutritional Information Per Serving: 375 calories, 23 grams fat, 13 grams protein, 3 grams fiber, 30 grams carbs

Time: 40 minutes prep, 1 hour total

Serving Size: 4 servings

Ingredients:

For the tofu batter:
- 14 ounces (1 package) tofu, extra firm
- ½ cup almond milk
- 1 tablespoon ground flaxseed
- 1 tablespoon flour
- 1 teaspoon white vinegar
- ½ teaspoon soy sauce
- ¼ teaspoon liquid smoke
- 1 teaspoon garlic, minced

For the crust:
- ½ cup flour
- ½ cup panko breadcrumbs
- ½ teaspoon paprika

- ½ teaspoon thyme
- ½ teaspoon Himalayan salt
- ¼ teaspoon black pepper

For the gravy:
- 1 tablespoon olive oil
- 1 onion, sliced
- ½ teaspoon dried thyme
- ¼ cup dry white wine
- 1 ½ tablespoon flour
- 1 cup vegetable broth
- 1 tablespoon soy sauce
- ½ teaspoon sugar

Directions:

1. Press the tofu using clean towels to remove as much water as possible. Set the wrapped tofu between heavy cookbooks to further drain the liquid.
2. To make the gravy, add olive oil, onion, thyme, and sugar to a non-stick skillet. Simmer over medium heat for 30 minutes, stirring occasionally.
3. After 30 minutes, add in the white wine and continue cooking until most of the liquid has evaporated.
4. Stir in the flour and stir to form a thick paste.

5. Stir in the broth and soy sauce. Cook for an additional 5 minutes until the gravy is thick. Set aside when finished.

6. To make the tofu steaks, whisk together all batter ingredients. Set aside for 10 minutes to allow thickening.

7. In a separate dish, mix all ingredients for the crust. Stir to incorporate.

8. Remove the tofu from the paper towels and slice the tofu in half widthwise. Then cut the tofu in half thickness-wise to create 4 steaks.

9. Heat a non-stick skillet with a dab of oil over medium heat.

10. Place the tofu into the batter, then coat evenly with the panko crust. Place the slab onto the skillet.

11. Cook each side of the tofu for 4 minutes. Be careful when flipping. The tofu should be golden brown.

12. Repeat steps 9 through 11 until no tofu remains.

13. Serve warm and pour the gravy over the steaks.

Dinner Recipe: Twenty

Meatloaf

Nutritional Information Per Serving: 286 calories, 7 grams fat, 14 grams protein, 10 grams fiber, 44 grams carbs

Time: 10 minutes prep, 1 hour total

Serving Size: 6 servings

Ingredients:

- 2 tablespoons olive oil
- 1 medium onion, finely chopped
- 2 small carrots, finely chopped
- 2 celery stalks, finely chopped
- 2 teaspoons garlic, minced
- 30 ounces (2 cans) chickpeas, drained and rinsed
- 1½ cups panko breadcrumbs
- 2 tablespoons ground flaxseed
- 3 tablespoons nutritional yeast
- 2 tablespoons soy sauce + 1 teaspoon soy sauce
- 2 tablespoons maple syrup, organic
- ¼ cup ketchup + ⅓ cup ketchup
- ½ teaspoon liquid smoke (optional)

- sea salt and black pepper to preference

Directions:

1. Preheat oven to 375°F. Lightly grease a 9-inch loaf pan or line with parchment paper.
2. Add onions, carrots, celery, garlic, and olive oil to a saucepan. Sauté over medium heat for 5 minutes. Set aside when finished.
3. In a large bowl, mash the chickpeas using a fork. Keep the texture thick and chunky.
4. Add the vegetables and all other ingredients (only 2 tablespoons soy sauce, ¼ cup ketchup) to the bowl containing the chickpeas. Stir until well combined.
5. Pour the mixture into the loaf pan. Push down and create an even surface.
6. Cover the loaf pan with foil and bake for 30 minutes.
7. **While the loaf cooks, whisk together the remaining ⅓ cup ketchup and 1 teaspoon of soy sauce in a small bowl for the sauce.**
8. When the loaf has baked for 30 minutes, remove and pour over sauce.
9. Return the loaf to the oven, uncovered, and bake for an additional 15 minutes.
10. Allow the loaf to rest for 15 minutes when done baking. Then slice and serve with additional ketchup and other sides.

Chapter 5:

Desserts

This section will take you through recipes for desserts. If you have a sweet tooth, you're in luck! Many desserts can still be healthy and satisfying at the same time. Vegan recipes aren't complicated, and great substitutes for your favorite ingredients have been discovered. Consider looking into a natural sweetener such as Stevia or monk fruit! You'll notice that these recipes typically call for maple syrup because, remember, honey is not considered a vegan food. Many bakery items that "require" eggs can be substituted using flax or applesauce. You'll notice this below, but it's also a great tip for adapting baked goodies using non-vegan recipes! Lastly, many of the recipes call for vegan, non-dairy chocolate chips. These are usually found in the health section in a grocery store.

Dessert Recipe: One

Grandma's Chocolate Chip Cookies

Nutritional Information Per Serving (1 Cookie): 160 calories, 7 grams fat, 2 grams protein, 1 grams fiber, 25 grams carbs

Time: 10 minutes prep, 20 minutes total

Serving Size: 24 cookies

Ingredients:

- 1 tablespoons ground flaxseed
- 2½ tablespoons water
- ½ cup vegan butter, softened
- 1¼ cups brown sugar
- 2 teaspoons vanilla extract
- 1½ cups all-purpose flour
- 2 teaspoons cornstarch
- 1 teaspoon baking soda
- ¼ teaspoon salt
- 1½ cups vegan chocolate chips (non-dairy)

Directions:

1. Prepare the flax egg by mixing flaxseed and water in a small bowl. Set aside to rest.

2. Preheat the oven to 350°F. Line 2 baking sheets with parchment paper.

3. Add butter to a medium bowl and beat for one minute using a hand mixer. The butter should be creamy.

4. Beat in the brown sugar and mix for 2 minutes until fluffy.

5. Add in the vanilla and flax egg.

6. Add 1 cup of flour, cornstarch, baking soda, and salt. Mix on low setting for 20 seconds.

7. Add in the rest of the flour. Mix until well combined. Do not over-mix.

8. Fold in the chocolate chips.

9. Using your hands, form the dough into a large ball.

10. Form the dough into small balls. Each cookie should use 1 to 2 tablespoons of dough each.

11. Place the dough onto the parchment paper and bake for 10 to 12 minutes. The edges should become golden brown.

12. Allow the cookies to cool for 5 minutes on the baking sheet then transfer to a cooling rack. Enjoy for up to 5 days.

Dessert Recipe: Two

Cinnamon Sugar Donuts

Nutritional Information Per Serving (1 Donut): 217 calories, 6 grams fat, 2 grams protein, 1 grams fiber, 38 grams carbs

Time: 10 minutes prep, 20 minutes total

Serving Size: 8 donuts

Ingredients:

- 1 cup all purpose flour
- ½ cup granulated sugar + ½ cup granulated sugar
- 1 teaspoon baking powder
- ¼ teaspoon salt
- ½ teaspoon cinnamon + 1 teaspoon cinnamon
- ½ cup and 2 tablespoons coconut milk, unsweetened
- 1 tablespoon applesauce
- 1 tablespoon coconut oil melted + ¼ cup coconut oil melted
- 1 teaspoon vanilla extract

Directions:

1. Preheat oven to 350°F. Lightly grease a donut pan.
2. In a bowl, whisk together flour, ½ cup sugar, baking powder, salt, and ½ teaspoon cinnamon.
3. Pour in coconut milk, applesauce, vanilla, and 1 tablespoon of melted coconut oil. Stir to incorporate. The batter should be thick, similar to a cake batter.
4. Fill the donut pan ¾ of the way full for each donut. The donuts will rise while baking.
5. Bake for 10 minutes.
6. Allow cooling for at least 3 minutes before removing the donuts. Transfer to a wire rack to cool further.
7. Prepare the glaze by placing ¼ cup melted coconut oil in a bowl. Set aside 1 teaspoon of cinnamon.
8. When the donuts have cooled, dip each donut into the oil, then sprinkle with cinnamon. Serve immediately afterwards.

Dessert Recipe: Three

Healthy Brownies

Nutritional Information Per Serving (1 Brownie):
78 calories, 2.5 grams fat, 3 grams protein, 3.5 grams fiber, 10 grams carbs

Time: 10 minutes prep, 1 hour and 10 minutes total

Serving Size: 16 servings

Ingredients:

For the brownies:
- ¾ cups dates (should be soft/moist)
- 1 teaspoon vanilla extract
- ⅓ cup and 1 tablespoon ground flax meal
- ¼ cup and 1 heaping teaspoon cocoa powder
- 4 tablespoons almond flour
- pinch of salt

For the glaze:
- ¼ cup maple syrup, organic
- 3 tablespoons peanut butter
- 4 tablespoons cocoa powder

Directions:

1. Line a 5-inch square baking pan with parchment paper. Use additional parchment paper for easy removal. Lightly grease.
2. To prepare the brownies, add flax meal, cocoa powder, pinch of salt, and almond flour to a food processor. Pulse a few times to well incorporate.
3. Add in dates and vanilla extract. Pulse to combine until a sticky dough forms. Add additional dates or a small amount of maple syrup as needed. The dough should stick to fingers when touching.
4. Transfer the dough into the lined baking dish.
5. Using your fingers, press down to create an even, firm surface.
6. In a small bowl, combine all glaze ingredients. Whisk until smooth.
7. Pour the glaze over the brownies.
8. Put the baking dish in the freezer for 1 hour.
9. Remove, thaw, and cut into 16 pieces. Store in the refrigerator or freezer.

Dessert Recipe: Four

Apple Crisp

Nutritional Information Per Serving: 375 calories, 15 grams fat, 7 grams protein, 3 grams fiber, 55 grams carbs

Time: 10 minutes prep, 45 minutes total

Serving Size: 9 servings

Ingredients:

For the filling:
- ¾ cup maple syrup, organic
- ½ cup almond butter
- ¼ teaspoon sea salt
- 2 medium red apples, peeled and chopped
- 1 teaspoon vanilla

For the topping:
- 2 cups rolled oats
- ½ cup almond butter
- ½ cup maple syrup, organic
- ½ teaspoon sea salt

Directions:

1. Preheat oven to 350°F. Set aside a medium-sized baking dish.
2. To prepare the filling, mix maple syrup, almond butter, and salt in a large bowl.
3. Add in apples and mix to incorporate.
4. Pour the filling into the baking dish.
5. To prepare the topping, add all ingredients to a food processor and pulse. The texture should remain chunky, with some oats remaining whole.
6. Pour the topping over the filling.
7. Bake for 35 minutes until the top begins to brown.
8. Serve warm with vegan whipped cream or vegan ice cream if desired.

Dessert Recipe: Five

Chocolate Mousse Cake

Nutritional Information Per Serving (1 Slice): 395 calories, 18 grams fat, 8 grams protein, 7 grams fiber, 50 grams carbs

Time: 30 minutes prep, 1 hour and 15 minutes total

Serving Size: 12 pieces

Ingredients:

For the cake:
- 1½ cup brown rice flour
- 1 cup coconut sugar
- ¾ cup cocoa powder, unsweetened
- 2 tablespoons ground flaxseed
- ¾ cup shredded dry coconut, unsweetened
- 2 teaspoons baking powder
- ¼ teaspoon baking soda
- ¼ teaspoon salt
- 2 cups zucchini, grated/lightly packed
- 1⅓ cup light coconut milk, canned
- 4 tablespoons maple syrup, organic

For the frosting:

- 2 small orange sweet potatoes, cooked
- 1 cup peanut butter, organic
- **⅓ cup maple syrup, organic**
- 4 tablespoons cocoa powder, unsweetened
- ¼ cup light coconut milk, canned
- ½ tablespoons vanilla extract
- pinch of salt

Directions:

1. Preheat oven to 375°F. Lightly grease and set aside an 8-inch springform cake pan.
2. Add all dry cake ingredients (everything except zucchini, coconut milk, and maple syrup) to a food processor. Pulse to incorporate, then pour into a large mixing bowl.
3. Slowly add in the coconut milk and maple syrup into the dry cake ingredients.
4. Stir in the grated zucchini with a spoon.
5. Pour batter into cake pan and bake for 40 to 45 minutes. A toothpick should come out clean when the center of the cake is pricked.
6. Allow the cake to cool in the pan for 30 minutes.
7. Cut the cake carefully in half to create a horizontal layer for the filling.
8. Add all frosting ingredients into a food processor. Start with a small amount of coconut milk and adjust until the frosting is thick.

9. Spread frosting on the bottom layer of the cake, then place the top layer over. Frost the outer portions of the cake.
10. Decorate with additional shredded coconut or vegan chocolate chips if desired. Store in the refrigerator for up to 5 days.

Dessert Recipe: Six

Four-Ingredient Peanut Butter Cookies

Nutritional Information Per Serving (1 Cookie): 265 calories, 18 grams fat, 9 grams protein, 2 grams fiber, 21 grams carbs

Time: 10 minutes prep, 22 minutes total

Serving Size: 8 cookies

Ingredients:

- 1 cup peanut butter
- ¾ cup oat flour
- ¼ cup and 1 tablespoon maple syrup
- 4 drops Stevia (optional)

Directions:

1. Preheat oven to 350°F and line a baking sheet with parchment paper.
2. Add peanut butter and maple syrup to a bowl.
3. Use a spatula and stir to form a paste.
4. Fold in the flour. A dough should begin to form.
5. Divide the dough into 8 equal parts.

6. Roll into balls and set each ball onto the cookie sheet. Flatten using a fork and leave an inch space between the cookies.

7. Bake for 16 minutes or until the sides are golden.

8. Allow the cookies to cool for at least 10 minutes on the tray, then transfer to a cooling rack. The cookies will harden over time.

9. Store in a glass jar for up to 2 weeks.

Dessert Recipe: Seven

Lemon Loaf

Nutritional Information Per Serving (1 Slice): 150 calories, 4 grams fat, 3 grams protein, 2 grams fiber, 28 grams carbs

Time: 10 minutes prep, 12 minutes total

Serving Size: 13 servings

Ingredients:

For the loaf:
- 2 cups oat flour
- 1 ½ teaspoon baking powder
- ¾ teaspoon salt
- ¼ teaspoon baking soda
- 1 cup sugar
- ¾ cup coconut milk
- ½ cup vegan yogurt
- ¼ cup coconut oil, melted
- ¼ cup lemon juice
- 1 tablespoon fresh lemon zest
- 1 teaspoon vanilla extract

For the glaze:

- ½ cup powdered sugar
- 1 tablespoon coconut milk

Directions:

1. Preheat oven to 350°F. Lightly grease a 9 x 5 inch loaf pan.
2. In a large bowl, combine all dry ingredients. Stir.
3. In a separate bowl, whisk all liquid ingredients.
4. Slowly combine the wet and dry ingredients. Stir as necessary to combine, but do not over-mix.
5. Pour mixture into loaf pan and smooth over to create an even top.
6. Bake for 50 to 55 minutes, until a toothpick comes out clean when the center of the loaf is pricked.
7. Allow the loaf to cool for 10 minutes in the loaf pan before transferring onto a cooling rack.
8. In a small bowl, whisk together powdered sugar and coconut milk.
9. Pour the glaze over the loaf and enjoy!

Dessert Recipe: Eight

Dark Chocolate Hummus

Nutritional Information Per Serving: 123 calories, 1 grams fat, 5 grams protein, 4 grams fiber, 23 grams carbs

Time: 5 minutes

Serving Size: 8 servings

Ingredients:

- 15 ounces (1 can) chickpeas, drained and rinsed
- ¼ cup cocoa powder
- ¼ cup maple syrup, organic
- 1 teaspoon vanilla extract
- ¼ teaspoon almond extract
- ¼ cup coconut milk

Directions:

1. Add all ingredients to a food processor and blend until smooth and creamy.
2. Garnish with a pinch of sea salt, vegan chocolate chips, or sliced almonds if desired. Best served with fruit or vegan graham crackers.

Dessert Recipe: Nine

Vanilla Coffee Cashew Ice Cream

Nutritional Information Per Serving: 290 calories, 18 grams fat, 7 grams protein, 2 grams fiber, 30 grams carbs

Time: 30 minutes (overnight recipe)

Serving Size: 6 servings

Ingredients:

- 1 cup brewed iced coffee
- 1 cup coconut milk, unsweetened
- 2 cups cashews, roasted and salted
- ½ cup maple syrup, organic
- 1 teaspoon vanilla extract

Directions:

1. Soak the cashews in the iced coffee and coconut milk overnight.
2. The following day, pour the coffee, coconut milk, and cashews into a blender.
3. Add all other ingredients to the blender. Blend until smooth and creamy.

4. Pour mixture into a parchment-lined loaf pan. Cover.

5. Freeze until firm. When ready to consume, allow 10 minutes of thawing beforehand.

Dessert Recipe: Ten

Chocolate Peanut Butter Cups

Nutritional Information Per Serving: 215 calories, 18 grams fat, 7 grams protein, 4 grams fiber, 9 grams carbs

Time: 15 minutes

Serving Size: 12 servings

Ingredients:

- ½ cup coconut butter
- 1 cup and 2 tablespoons peanut butter, organic
- 5 tablespoons cocoa powder, unsweetened
- Stevia drops to preference (optional)

Directions:

1. Line 12 muffin tin cups with aluminum cupcake liners.
2. Add the coconut butter to a microwave-safe bowl and heat in 10-second intervals until melted.
3. Add in peanut butter and cocoa powder. Whisk until smooth. Add Stevia, if using.
4. Distribute the batter evenly into the liners (about 2 tablespoons each).

5. Put the muffin pan into the freezer for 20 minutes or until firm.

6. Store in the refrigerator for up to 2 weeks.

Chapter 6:

Snacks

Snacks are a great way to keep your body full throughout the day, and these recipes will help you make sure you're eating nutritious and delicious ones. As a bodybuilder, your metabolism is likely running all day, every day, at a fast pace. Many of the snack recipes given below will give you the energy and nutrients your body needs to recover. These options will satisfy any sweet tooth or salty snack lover!

Snack Recipe: One

Seeded Crackers

Nutritional Information Per Serving (1 Cracker): 26 calories, 2 grams fat, 1 grams protein, 1 grams fiber, 2 grams carbs

Time: 10 minutes prep, 1 hour total

Serving Size: 36 crackers

Ingredients:

- ½ cup pumpkin seeds
- ½ cup sunflower seeds
- ¼ cup sesame seeds
- ¼ cup chia seeds
- ¾ cup water
- ¾ teaspoon salt
- 1 teaspoon rosemary
- 1 teaspoon onion powder

Directions:

1. Preheat oven to 350°F. Set aside two large pieces of parchment paper.
2. Combine all ingredients in a large bowl. Set aside to rest for 15 minutes.

3. Oil one side of each of the two sheets of parchment paper to avoid sticking in the next step.
4. Place the dough between the two pieces of parchment paper. Roll out the dough thin using a rolling pin (roll to approximately 10 x 14 inch rectangle).
5. Slide the rolled out dough onto a baker's half sheet.
6. Bake for 20 minutes.
7. Remove from oven and cut into large pieces. Flip each piece over when finished.
8. Bake for an additional 14 minutes.
9. Let cool and store in an airtight container.

Snack Recipe: Two

Banana Bites

Nutritional Information Per Serving: 273 calories, 14 grams fat, 6 grams protein, 5 grams fiber, 37 grams carbs

Time: 15 minutes prep, 15 minutes total

Serving Size: 4 servings

Ingredients:

- 2 bananas
- ½ cup vegan chocolate, melted
- 1 cup roasted pistachios, in pieces or finely crushed

Directions:

1. Set aside a parchment-lined baking sheet.
2. Peel the bananas and stick a toothpick in both ends to make the next step easier.
3. Dip and fully coat the bananas in the melted chocolate. Set onto the parchment paper.
4. If using whole pistachios, place the nuts into a food processor and pulse until fine. Leave some pistachios intact.

5. Sprinkle the pistachios on top of the banana.

6. Freeze the bananas to set the chocolate and pistachios for 5 minutes.

7. Remove the bananas and cut into bites. Return to the freezer in a glass container.

8. When ready to consume, remove bananas from the freezer and thaw for 10 minutes to soften.

Snack Recipe: Three

Plantain Chips

Nutritional Information Per Serving: 200 calories, 10 grams fat, 2 grams protein, 3 grams fiber, 30 grams carbs

Time: 15 minutes prep, 35 minutes total

Serving Size: 4 servings

Ingredients:

- 2 green (slightly yellow) plantains, washed and peeled
- ½ tablespoon onion powder
- ½ tablespoon paprika
- ½ teaspoon salt
- 1½ tablespoon avocado oil

Directions:

1. Preheat the oven to 350°F.
2. Cut the plantains into very thin slices using a sharp knife. Place the slices into a medium mixing bowl.
3. In a small bowl, whisk together all the spices and avocado oil. Pour mixture into the bowl

containing the plantains. Mix until well incorporated.

4. Place plantains onto a large non-stick baking sheet.

5. Bake for 20 minutes.

6. Remove and let cool before storing in an airtight container.

Snack Recipe: Four

Homemade Hummus

Nutritional Information Per Serving: 330 calories, 17 grams fat, 12 grams protein, 9 grams fiber, 35 grams carbs

Time: 3 minutes

Serving Size: 8 servings

Ingredients:

- 30 ounces (2 cans) garbanzo beans
- ⅓ cup chickpea liquid
- ½ cup tahini
- ¼ cup olive oil
- 2 lemons, juiced
- 2 teaspoons garlic, minced
- ½ teaspoon salt

Directions:

1. Add all ingredients to a blender. Blend until smooth for about 30 seconds.
2. Transfer to an airtight container and sprinkle with additional seasonings or olive oil if desired.

Snack Recipe: Five

Spinach and Artichoke Dip

Nutritional Information Per Serving: 75 calories, 6 grams fat, 3 grams protein, 6 grams fiber, 5 grams carbs

Time: 10 minutes prep, 20 minutes total

Serving Size: 10 servings

Ingredients:

- 1 tablespoon olive oil
- 2 teaspoons garlic, minced
- 12 ounces marinated artichoke hearts
- 4 cups baby spinach, roughly chopped
- ¼ cup vegan mayonnaise
- 8 ounces vegan cream cheese
- ½ teaspoon onion powder
- ½ teaspoon salt

Directions:

1. Preheat the oven to 400°F.
2. Add olive oil, garlic, artichoke hearts, and spinach to skillet. Sauté for about 3 minutes to soften the vegetables.

3. Add cream cheese, mayo, and spices. Mix until well incorporated.
4. Add the mixture to an oven-safe baking dish. Broil for 5 minutes.
5. Remove from the oven and serve warm with crackers or chips. This recipe is great to bring to social events.

Snack Recipe: Six

Curry White Bean Cup

Nutritional Information Per Serving: 280 calories, 14 grams of fat, 12 grams protein, 8 grams of fiber, 32 grams carbs

Time: 10 minutes

Serving Size: 4 servings

Ingredients:

- 1 can white beans
- 1 garlic clove
- 1 tablespoon lemon juice
- ¼ cup avocado oil
- 3 teaspoons curry powder
- ½ teaspoon paprika
- sea salt and black pepper to preference

Directions:

1. Add all ingredients to a food processor and blend until smooth.
2. Transfer to an airtight container and store in the refrigerator until ready to be consumed.

Snack Recipe: Seven

Vegan Onion Rings

Nutritional Information Per Serving: 200 calories, 1 grams fat, 6 grams protein, 3 grams fiber, 40 grams carbs

Time: 10 minutes prep, 30 minutes total

Serving Size: 4 servings

Ingredients:

- 2 sweet onions, peeled
- ⅔ cup all-purpose flour
- ⅔ cup almond milk, unsweetened
- 1 teaspoon garlic powder
- 1 teaspoon smoked paprika powder
- 1 tablespoon nutritional yeast
- 1 cup panko breadcrumbs
- ¼ teaspoon salt

Directions:

1. Preheat oven to 350°F. Line a baking sheet with parchment paper.
2. Combine flour, spices, nutritional yeast, and almond milk in a bowl. Stir well.

3. Place the breadcrumbs into a separate bowl.

4. Cut the onions into ¼ inch rings and separate.

5. Coat each onion ring in the spices, then follow by dipping in the breadcrumbs.Lay the onion rings onto the baking sheet when finished.

6. Bake for 20 minutes.

7. Remove the pan and flip each onion ring. Bake for an additional 10 minutes.

8. Serve warm with additional dipping sauce if desired.

Snack Recipe: Eight

Roasted Chickpeas

Nutritional Information Per Serving: 265 calories, 11 grams fat, 11 grams protein, 10 grams fiber, 30 grams carbs

Time: 5 minutes prep, 40 minutes total

Serving Size: 4 servings

Ingredients:

- 30 ounces (2 cans) chickpeas, drained and rinsed
- 2 tablespoons avocado oil
- 1 teaspoon smoked paprika powder
- 1 teaspoon onion powder
- ½ teaspoon salt

Directions:

1. Preheat the oven to 350°F. Line a baking sheet with parchment paper.
2. Use a clean dish towel to gently squeeze out any water left on the chickpeas. You'll want them as dry as possible.

3. Add the chickpeas to a bowl and toss in the avocado oil.

4. Spread the chickpeas out on the baking sheet.

5. Bake for 25 minutes.

6. Remove chickpeas from the oven and place in the bowl used before. Toss in all spices and shake until well combined.

7. Return the chickpeas to the baking sheet and bake for an additional 10 minutes. The chickpeas should turn golden brown.

8. Store in an airtight container once cooled.

Snack Recipe: Nine

Protein Balls

Nutritional Information Per Serving (1 Ball): 130 calories, 9 grams fat, 5 grams protein, 4 grams fiber, 11 grams carbs

Time: 10 minutes

Serving Size: 16 protein balls

Ingredients:

- ½ cup peanut butter, organic
- ½ cup ground flaxseed
- 1 cup rolled oats
- 2 tablespoons maple syrup, organic
- ¼ cup vegan or non-dairy chocolate chips

Directions:

1. Combine all ingredients in a bowl. Stir to incorporate.
2. Use an ice cream scooper to divide the dough into 16 balls. Roll and place into an airtight container.
3. Store in the refrigerator for up to 5 days.

Snack Recipe: Ten

Guacamole

Nutritional Information Per Serving: 110 calories, 10 grams fat, 1.5 grams protein, 4 grams fiber, 6 grams carbs

Time: 10 minutes

Serving Size: 8 servings

Ingredients:

- 2 avocados, ripe
- 1 tablespoon lime juice
- 1 cup cilantro, roughly chopped
- ½ cup red onion, roughly chopped
- ½ cup cherry tomatoes, quartered (optional)
- ¼ cup canned jalapeño peppers, chopped
- ¼ teaspoon garlic powder
- ¼ teaspoon cumin
- ½ teaspoon salt

Directions:

1. Add onion, tomato, jalapeño peppers, and lime juice to a mixing bowl. Sprinkle in all seasonings and stir to incorporate.

2. Fold in avocado chunks. Stir, but do not over-mix, to create a thick texture.

3. Serve immediately over a salad, as a side, with vegetables, or with crackers.

Snack Recipe: Eleven

Banana Bread

Nutritional Information Per Serving: 120 calories, 0.5 grams fat, 2.5 grams protein, 1.5 grams fiber, 27 grams carbs

Time: 10 minutes prep, 1 hour and 5 minutes total

Serving Size: 12 servings

Ingredients:

- 3 bananas, ripe
- ⅓ cup applesauce, unsweetened
- ¼ cup almond milk
- 1 teaspoon vanilla extract
- 1¾ cup whole wheat flour
- ⅓ cup coconut sugar
- 2 teaspoons baking powder
- ½ teaspoon baking soda
- ⅓ cup chopped walnuts
- ¼ teaspoon salt

Directions:

1. Preheat oven to 350°F. Line a 9-inch loaf pan with parchment paper.

2. In a medium bowl, mash bananas until smooth. Add applesauce, vanilla, and almond milk and mix well.
3. Add in all other ingredients. Stir, but do not over-process.
4. Pour batter into loaf pan. Use a spatula to smooth the top.
5. Bake for 50 to 55 minutes. A toothpick should come out clean when the center is pricked.

Snack Recipe: Twelve

Mint Shake

Nutritional Information Per Serving: 130 calories, 7 grams fat, 1.5 grams protein, 3 grams fiber, 16 grams carbs

Time: 5 minutes prep, 10 minutes total

Serving Size: 2 servings

Ingredients:

- 1 cup coconut milk
- ¼ avocado
- 1 banana, frozen
- ½ cup baby spinach
- ⅛ teaspoon peppermint extract
- ½ teaspoon vanilla extract
- 1 tablespoon vegan chocolate chips

Directions:

1. Add all ingredients to a blender, excluding the chocolate chips. Blend until smooth.
2. Pulse in chocolate chips or sprinkle over the shake once poured into a glass.
3. Serve immediately.

Snack Recipe: Thirteen

Salt and Vinegar Chips

Nutritional Information Per Serving: 13 calories, 1 grams fat, 0.5 grams protein, 0.5 grams fiber, 0 grams carbs

Time: 10 minutes prep, 12 hours and 10 minutes total

Serving Size: 8 servings

Ingredients:

- 1 zucchini
- 2 teaspoons of olive oil, extra virgin
- 2 tablespoons apple cider vinegar
- Himalayan salt to preference

Directions:

1. Preheat oven to 110°F.
2. Use a mandoline to slice the zucchini very thin. Turn the setting to ⅛. A knife can also be used carefully if you do not own a mandoline.
3. Add the zucchini to a bowl and toss in all other ingredients.
4. Pour the zucchini onto teflon-lined sheets.
5. Bake and dehydrate for 12 hours until crispy.

Snack Recipe: Fourteen

Black Bean Dip

Nutritional Information Per Serving: 70 calories, 0.5 grams fat, 5 grams protein, 4 grams fiber, 13 grams carbs

Time: 5 minutes prep, 15 minutes total

Serving Size: 6 servings

Ingredients:

- 15 ounces (1 can) black beans, drained and rinsed
- 2 tablespoons red onion, roughly chopped
- 1 small tomato, chopped
- 2 teaspoons garlic, minced
- ½ teaspoon cumin
- ½ lime, juiced
- Himalayan salt to preference

Directions:

1. Add all ingredients to a food processor and pulse until combined.
2. Serve hot or warm. This recipe also makes a great dressing for salads.

Snack Recipe: Fifteen

Easy Stovetop Bread

Nutritional Information Per Serving: 165 calories, 8 grams fat, 4 grams protein, 3 grams fiber, 23 grams carbs

Time: 10 minutes prep, 15 minutes total

Serving Size: 4 servings

Ingredients:

- 1 cup all-purpose flour
- 1 teaspoon baking powder
- 2 tablespoons olive oil
- ½ teaspoon salt
- ⅓ cup warm water
- ½ teaspoon rosemary
- ½ teaspoon herbs of choice

Directions:

1. In a mixing bowl, combine flour, baking powder, and salt.
2. Stir in olive oil and water. Stir until combined, but do not over-process.

3. Lightly coat a skillet with olive oil and warm over medium heat.
4. Shape the dough into 4 patties.
5. Drop the dough into the skillet. Cook each side for 5 minutes.
6. Sprinkle herbs on each side while cooking.
7. Serve immediately or microwave when ready to consume.

Chapter 7:

Workout Fuel

This chapter will take you through what to eat before and after a workout. However, because everyone is different, taking a bit of time to figure out what's best for you will help you achieve your fitness goals faster.

As a general rule of thumb, it's not best to eat immediately before a workout. The body will put more energy toward digesting food instead of supporting muscle contraction during your workout. You may also experience discomfort while training if you have eaten something large beforehand. Eating one to three hours before a workout is suggested. This will regulate your blood sugars, keep you from feeling hungry, and fuel your muscles, which will overall lead to a better workout. A larger meal should be consumed five to six hours before exercising. Avoid foods high in fiber directly before a workout, as it can lead to a feeling of heaviness and discomfort.

For strength training, pre-workout meals should include low glycemic carbs and protein-rich foods. Low glycemic carbs are typically lower in sugar, and can include whole grains, certain vegetables, nuts, and seeds. For a cardio session, you should consume more carbs than proteins before the work out. The carbs will give you energy and metabolize fast giving quick bursts of energy suitable for high-intensity cardio. Starchy foods like bread, rice, pasta, or fruits are suitable. Stick to lower glycemic carbs or less sugary foods for a long cardio session, as your body needs more sustained energy releases.

After a workout, it's important to replenish the nutrients lost. Both carbs and protein should be consumed. This will help your muscles recover, repair, and rebuild. The process where your body recovers from an intense workout session begins directly after and lasts for a while, depending on the activities performed. Strength training requires a longer recovery, while cardio recovery takes place at a quicker rate. It's important to fuel this process so the body can do its job efficiently. Consume a quick snack or meal directly after. If you work out in the evening, it's possible you will need an additional snack before bed as well, to aid in the process overnight. Remember to drink a lot of water to stay hydrated before, during, and after.

Pre-Workout Recipe: One

Chocolate Pudding

Nutritional Information Per Serving: 560 calories, 30 grams fat, 11 grams protein, 12 grams fiber, 25 grams carbs

Time: 5 minutes

Serving Size: 4 servings

Ingredients:

- 2 avocados, ripe
- 1 banana
- ½ cup cocoa powder, unsweetened
- ½ cup natural peanut butter
- 2 tablespoons maple syrup

Directions:

1. Add all ingredients to a blender and blend until creamy. Add a few drops of water as necessary to help blend.
2. Serve immediately or store in the refrigerator.

Pre-Workout Recipe: Two

Coconut Bites

Nutritional Information Per Serving (1 Bite): 150 calories, 12 grams fat, 4 grams protein, 4 grams fiber, 8 grams carbs

Time: 30 minutes

Serving Size: 20 servings

Ingredients:

- 1½ cups shredded coconut, unsweetened
- 1½ cups almond flour
- 2 tablespoons flax meal
- 3 tablespoons hemp seeds
- 2 tablespoons vegan protein powder
- ⅓ cup tahini
- 4 tablespoons coconut butter
- ¼ cup cocoa powder
- ¼ teaspoon cinnamon
- 3 pitted dates
- pinch of salt

Directions:

1. Line a baking sheet with parchment paper.

2. Add all ingredients to a food processor. Blend
    for 3 to 5 minutes until a paste forms.
3. Add more coconut butter if the mixture is too
    dry. Add more coconut shreds if the batter is
    too thick.
4. Scoop out 2-tablespoon-sized bites. Place onto
    parchment paper.
5. Place the balls in the refrigerator once done and
    store for up to a week.

Pre-Workout Recipe: Three

Nut Butter Toast

Nutritional Information Per Serving: 450 calories, 27 grams fat, 19 grams protein, 10 grams fiber, 40 grams carbs

Time: 5 minutes

Serving Size: 1 serving

Ingredients:

- 2 slices Ezekiel bread or seeded bread, toasted
- 2 tablespoons almond butter
- 2 tablespoons hulled hemp seeds

Directions:

1. Spread the nut butter onto the toast.
2. Sprinkle hemp seeds over the toast. Enjoy warm.

Pre-Workout Recipe: Four

Blueberry Smoothie

Nutritional Information Per Serving: 218 calories, 10 grams fat, 6.5 grams protein, 5 grams fiber, 31 grams carbs

Time: 5 minutes

Serving Size: 2 servings

Ingredients:

- 1 large banana, frozen
- 1 cup organic blueberries, frozen
- 1 stalk celery
- ⅔ cup zucchini, sliced
- handful of spinach
- 1 tablespoon hemp seeds
- ¼ teaspoon cinnamon
- 1 cup light coconut milk
- ½ teaspoon maca powder

Directions:

1. Add all ingredients to a blender and blend until smooth. Enjoy immediately.

Pre-Workout Recipe: Five

Morning Metabolism Boost Water

Nutritional Information Per Serving: 22 calories, 0 grams fat, 0 grams protein, 1 grams fiber, 6 grams carbs

Time: 2 minutes

Serving Size: 1 serving

Ingredients:

- 4 inch piece ginger, sliced
- 4 cups water
- pinch of cinnamon
- ½ lemon, juiced
- 1 tablespoon apple cider vinegar
- pinch of cayenne pepper

Directions:

1. Add all ingredients to a glass jar or cup. Shake or stir until evenly mixed.

Pre-Workout Recipe: Six

PB & J Stuffed Dates

Nutritional Information Per Serving: 165 calories, 8 grams fat, 4 grams protein, 3 grams fiber, 23 grams carbs

Time: 5 minutes prep, 30 minutes total

Serving Size: 12 dates

Ingredients:

- 12 medjool dates
- ¼ cup peanut butter, organic
- 1 cup raspberries
- 1 teaspoon chia seeds
- 2 tablespoons maple syrup
- pinch of salt
- 2 tablespoons vegan dark chocolate chips

Directions:

1. Add raspberries to a saucepan and turn to medium heat. Cook for 5 minutes and stir occasionally.
2. Use a wooden spoon to muddle the raspberries.

3. Add chia seeds, maple syrup, and a pinch of salt.

4. Simmer the jam for 2 more minutes, stirring occasionally.

5. Leave the jam to sit for 10 minutes.

6. Prepare the dates by slicing each vertically. Remove pits.

7. Fill each date with 1 teaspoon of peanut butter and 1 teaspoon of jam.

8. Sprinkle chocolate chips over the dates. Store extras in the refrigerator.

Pre-Workout Recipe: Seven

Trail Mix

Nutritional Information Per Serving: 403 calories, 26 grams fat, 8 grams protein, 4 grams fiber, 37 grams carbs

Time: 5 minutes

Serving Size: 6 serving

Ingredients:

- 1 cup macadamia nuts
- ½ cup almonds
- ½ cups pistachios
- ½ cup cherries
- ½ cup cranberries
- ¼ cup vegan chocolate chips

Directions:

1. Mix all ingredients in an airtight, resealable bag and store.

Pre-Workout Recipe: Eight

Strawberry and Banana Smoothie Bowl

Nutritional Information Per Serving: 639 calories, 13 grams fat, 14 grams protein, 19 grams fiber, 126 grams carbs

Time: 5 minutes

Serving Size: 1 serving

Ingredients:

- 3 large bananas
- ¼ cup rolled oats
- ½ cup organic strawberries
- ½ cup cooked chickpeas
- 1 tablespoon almond butter
- ¼ cup coconut milk
- toppings of choice

Directions:

1. Put all ingredients except desired toppings into a high-speed blender. Blend until smooth.
2. Pour the smoothie into a bowl and add toppings such as additional fruit, almond flakes, goji berries, or dark chocolate chunks.

Pre-Workout Recipe: Nine

Mango Pops

Nutritional Information Per Serving: 189 calories, 12 grams fat, 2 grams protein, 5 grams fiber, 20 grams carbs

Time: 5 minutes

Serving Size: 2 servings

Ingredients:

- ½ cup mango, frozen
- ½ cup pineapple, frozen
- 1 scoop vanilla vegan protein
- 14 ounces (1 can) canned light coconut milk

Directions:

1. Place all ingredients into a blender. Blend until smooth.
2. Pour the mixture into popsicle molds. Freeze.
3. When ready to consume, allow the popsicles to thaw for 5 or 10 minutes.

Pre-Workout Recipe: Ten

Pistachio Energy Bites

Nutritional Information Per Serving: 115 calories, 2 grams fat, 4 grams protein, 2 grams fiber, 3 grams carbs

Time: 5 minutes prep, 10 minutes total

Serving Size: 10 servings

Ingredients:

- ½ cup raw pistachios, shelled/unsalted
- 1 cup pitted dates
- ½ cup chia seeds

Directions:

1. Add half of the pistachios to a food processor and process until a powder appears. Pour into a bowl when finished.
2. Add remaining ingredients to the food processor. Process until a spongy dough appears.
3. Using your hands or a cookie scoop, roll the dough into small balls.
4. Roll the balls into the crushed pistachio.

5. Place the balls into an airtight container and
    store in the refrigerator for up to 7 days.

Post-Workout Recipe: One

Pea Soup

Nutritional Information Per Serving: 143 calories, 6 grams fat, 9 grams protein, 6.5 grams fiber, 16 grams carbs

Time: 5 minutes prep, 30 minutes total

Serving Size: 4 servings

Ingredients:

- 2 tablespoons olive oil, more as needed
- 12 ounces (1 large bundle) asparagus, trimmed
- 2 cups peas
- 4 cloves garlic, minced
- 1 medium shallot, thinly sliced
- 1½ cup almond milk, unsweetened
- 1½ cup vegetable broth
- 2 tablespoons nutritional yeast
- ½ lemon, juiced
- Himalayan salt and black pepper to preference

Directions:

1. Preheat the oven to 400°F.

2. Place the asparagus onto a baking sheet. Drizzle with olive oil, and sprinkle with salt and pepper.
3. Roast the asparagus for 15 minutes. Set aside when finished.
4. Add olive oil to a large soup pot over medium heat. Add shallot and garlic and sprinkle in salt and pepper. Simmer for 3 minutes.
5. Add in peas, vegetable broth, and almond milk. Stir.
6. Transfer the mixture to a blender, along with the asparagus. Work in batches if needed. Blend until smooth and transfer back to the pot.
7. Whisk in nutritional yeast.
8. Bring the soup to a boil, then reduce to low heat. Simmer for 5 minutes.
9. Remove from heat and stir in lemon juice. Serve warm.

Post-Workout Recipe: Two

Green Smoothie

Nutritional Information Per Serving: 330 calories, 2 grams fat, 18 grams protein, 13 grams fiber, 68 grams carbs

Time: 5 minutes

Serving Size: 1 serving

Ingredients:

- 2 cups kale, stems removed
- 1 apple, sliced
- 2 celery stalks
- ½ banana
- 1 cup parsley
- ½ cup blueberries
- 1 inch ginger root, roughly chopped
- ½ teaspoon cinnamon
- 1 scoop vegan protein powder
- 1 cup lemon juice
- ice

Directions:

1. Add all ingredients to a blender and blend until smooth. Add ice and water as needed to reach desired consistency.

Post-Workout Recipe: Three

Roasted Red Pepper Hummus

Nutritional Information Per Serving: 135 calories, 8 grams fat, 4 grams protein, 3 grams fiber, 11 grams carbs

Time: 5 minutes prep, 30 minutes total

Serving Size: 8 servings

Ingredients:

- 2 red peppers
- 2 tablespoons olive oil, more as needed
- 15 ounces (1 can) garbanzo beans
- ¼ cup tahini
- ¼ cup lemon juice
- 1 clove garlic, minced
- ¼ cup water
- sea salt and black pepper to preference

Directions:

1. Preheat oven to 450°F.
2. Slice the red pepper in half and remove the seeds.

3. Drizzle olive oil over interior and exterior of the red pepper.
4. Place the peppers into the oven, skin side facing up. Roast for 25 minutes or until charred.
5. Remove the skin after the pepper are cooled.
6. Add all ingredients to a food processor and blend until smooth.
7. Serve chilled with crackers, over a salad, or on a sandwich for extra nutrients.

Post-Workout Recipe: Four

Superfood Salad

Nutritional Information Per Serving: 800 calories, 49 grams fat, 20 grams protein, 22 grams fiber, 81 grams carbs

Time: 5 minutes prep, 30 minutes total

Serving Size: 4 servings

Ingredients:

For the salad:
- 1 cup red quinoa, uncooked
- 2 teaspoons of olive oil
- 2 cups sweet potato, diced
- 14 ounces (1 can) chickpeas, drained and rinsed
- 2 cups arugula
- 2 cups cherry tomatoes, halved
- 2 avocados, pitted
- 4 tablespoons pepitas

For the sauce:
- 2 cups cashews
- 1 ¼ cup water
- 2 cloves garlic

- 1 teaspoon salt
- Sriracha to preference

Directions:

1. To make the sauce, pour hot water over the cashews. Allow them to soak for as long as possible while the salad is being prepared. Drain afterwards.
2. Add all the sauce ingredients to a blender and blend until smooth. Add water as needed to reach desired consistency.
3. Cook the quinoa using the instructions on the packaging.
4. Add a teaspoon of olive oil to a skillet over medium heat.
5. Once oil is warmed, add the sweet potato chunks and cook for 3 minutes. Stir frequently to prevent burning.
6. Add another teaspoon of oil to the skillet and add in chickpeas. Sauté for 4 minutes. The chickpeas should be toasted and the sweet potatoes tender. Turn off the heat and set aside when finished.
7. Divide the quinoa into 4 bowls. Divide the remaining ingredients.
8. Drizzle over the sauce and serve immediately.

Post-Workout Recipe: Five

Fresh Pesto Pasta

Nutritional Information Per Serving: 620 calories, 41 grams fat, 16 grams protein, 7 grams fiber, 55 grams carbs

Time: 20 minutes prep, 30 minutes total

Serving Size: 4 servings

Ingredients:

For the pasta:
- 8 ounces pasta
- 2 cups cherry tomatoes
- 2 cups asparagus, chopped
- 2 cups mushrooms, sliced
- 3 cloves garlic
- 1 teaspoon olive oil
- sea salt and black pepper to preference

For the sauce:
- 1 cup walnuts
- 1½ cup basil leaves
- ¼ cup olive oil
- ½ teaspoon garlic, minced

- ½ lemon, juiced
- sea salt and black pepper to preference

Directions:

1. Preheat the oven to 425°F.
2. Cook the pasta using the directions on the packaging. Drain when finished and place the pasta back into a large pot.
3. To prepare the pasta ingredients, arrange the vegetables on a baking pan. Sprinkle over olive oil and salt.
4. Peel the garlic cloves and place in a small piece of aluminum foil. Drizzle with a small amount of olive oil before wrapping up. Place it on the same baking pan.
5. Roast the vegetables for 25 minutes.
6. Remove the garlic from the aluminum foil and use a fork to mash. It should form a paste.
7. To make the sauce, place all the sauce ingredients into a food processor. Pulse until smooth.
8. When all the elements are finished, add everything to the pot containing the pasta. Stir until well combined.
9. Let the pasta simmer over low heat for a few minutes to warm and combine the pasta further. Serve immediately or chilled.

Post-Workout Recipe: Six

Chia Seed Pudding

Nutritional Information Per Serving: 255 calories, 14 grams fat, 8 grams protein, 12 grams fiber, 26 grams carbs

Time: 5 minutes prep, 20 minutes total (overnight recipe)

Serving Size: 2 servings

Ingredients:

- ½ cup blueberries
- 1 cup coconut milk, unsweetened
- 1 teaspoon vanilla extract
- 1 teaspoon cinnamon
- 1 tablespoon maple syrup
- 1 tablespoon hemp seeds
- ⅓ cup chia seeds

Directions:

1. Place blueberries, coconut milk, vanilla, cinnamon, hemp seeds, and maple syrup in a blender. Process until smooth.
2. Pour mixture into a large canning jar or bowl.

3. Stir in chia seeds.

4. Leave the mixture to rest overnight in the refrigerator.

5. The following day, top with additional toppings like nuts or fruit before serving.

Post-Workout Recipe: Seven

Veggie Wrap

Nutritional Information Per Serving: 360 calories, 17 grams fat, 14 grams protein, 11 grams fiber, 20 grams carbs

Time: 5 minutes

Serving Size: 3 servings

Ingredients:

- 6 leaves romaine lettuce
- ½ cucumber, sliced
- ½ red pepper, sliced
- 1 avocado, pitted
- ¾ cup hummus of choice
- 2 tablespoons olive oil
- 2 tortillas

Directions:

1. Evenly distribute all ingredients onto each tortilla. Serve immediately.

Post-Workout Recipe: Eight

Avocado Pesto Panini

Nutritional Information Per Serving: 710 calories, 52 grams fat, 2 grams protein, 7 grams fiber, 58 grams carbs

Time: 5 minutes prep, 10 minutes total

Serving Size: 1 serving

Ingredients:

For the sandwich:
- 2 slices seeded bread
- 3 slices vegan mozzarella
- ½ avocado, in 4 slices
- 4 teaspoons vegan mayo

For the sauce:
- 1 ½ cups fresh basil
- ½ avocado
- 1 tablespoon lemon juice
- ½ teaspoon garlic powder
- 1 teaspoon olive oil
- 1 tablespoon pine nuts
- 1 tablespoon nutritional yeast

- sea salt to preference

Directions:

1. To make the sauce, place all ingredients into a blender and blend until smooth.
2. Assemble the sandwich by spreading the sauce on 1 side of each bread slice.
3. Add mozzarella and avocado to the sandwich. Close the sandwich.
4. Spread ½ of the vegan mayonnaise on the bottom slice of the sandwich. Then place onto a skillet.
5. While one side cooks, spread the mayo on the side of the bread that's facing you.
6. Flip the sandwich and cook both sides until golden brown and toasty.

Post-Workout Recipe: Nine

Enchilada Bowl

Nutritional Information Per Serving: 280 calories, 7 grams fat, 10 grams protein, 9 grams fiber, 45 grams carbs

Time: 5 minutes prep, 35 minutes total

Serving Size: 6 servings

Ingredients:

For the bowl:
- 1 cup quinoa, cooked
- 1 cup onion, chopped
- 2 tablespoons olive oil
- 1 cup red pepper, chopped
- 15 ounces (1 can) black beans
- 1 cup corn

For the sauce:
- 15 ounces (1 can) tomato sauce
- 1 teaspoon chili powder
- 1 teaspoon cumin
- 1 teaspoon garlic powder
- 1 teaspoon onion powder

- 1 teaspoon oregano
- ¼ cup vegetable broth

Directions:

1. Add olive oil to a skillet over medium heat. After 30 seconds, add in onions. Cook for 2 minutes, then add in red peppers.
2. To prepare the sauce, combine all sauce ingredients in a saucepan. Bring the contents to a boil, then reduce to low heat. Simmer for 5 minutes.
3. Assemble the bowls by placing in quinoa, vegetables, beans, and corn. Pour the sauce over the top. Serve with vegan sour cream, guacamole, or hot sauce if desired.

Post-Workout Recipe: Ten

Spicy Hummus Pizza

Nutritional Information Per Serving: 185 calories, 5 grams fat, 7 grams protein, 5 grams fiber, 28 grams carbs

Time: 5 minutes prep, 17 minutes total

Serving Size: 1 serving

Ingredients:

- 1 large whole wheat tortillas.
- 2 tablespoons red pepper hummus
- 3 tablespoons marinara sauce
- ½ tomato, sliced
- 1 tablespoon sliced onion
- 1 tablespoon nutritional yeast
- red pepper flakes to preference (optional)

Directions:

1. Preheat oven to 325°F.
2. Bake the tortilla for 3 minutes until crispy.
3. Spread the hummus on top of the tortilla. Spread marinara over the top.

4. Add all other ingredients on top, excluding the nutritional yeast.

5. Bake for an additional 4 minutes.

6. Sprinkle nutritional yeast and any other desired sauce.

Conclusion

Now that you have read through this guide, it's time to enjoy some of the wonderful recipes found within. You have all the tools you'll need to begin or continue reaching for your fitness and health goals. Deciding to embark on a vegan lifestyle is the best decision you can make for the environment, animals, and your personal health. As technology advances, the studies surrounding the animal product industry are alarming. Additionally, regular consumption of meat is linked to cancer, cardiovascular disease, diabetes, chronic illnesses, and obesity. Consuming meat has a clear effect on health, as many meats have been classified as a type one carcinogen. Behind closed doors, animals are being subjected to harsh environments, tight living quarters, fecal matter, and disease. Even when meat receives the organic label, the internal health of the animal does not have to be disclosed. On top of this, the environment is suffering greatly. Remember that, as mentioned before, a car would have to drive 200 miles to produce the same amount of emissions as a single burger containing a half-pound of meat. Rainforest destruction and land clearing is disrupting natural habitats and the ecosystem that supports our planet. Water is becoming polluted from animal waste and becoming increasingly scarce as producers try to hydrate copious numbers of animals.

Deciding to go vegan for any of the above reasons is the right choice. Your body will thank you and will become healthier and stronger than before. Being a bodybuilder lies on the basic principles of balancing your macronutrients and micronutrients. Consuming the right amounts of each—from nutritious sources—will support muscle mass and reduce your carbon footprint. With the information from this book, you'll be able to identify important nutrients and their functions. While fitness goals are great, keeping a healthy, strong body on the inside is just as important. Remember that the macro guidelines offered can be adjusted to help you get started and can be modified as you meet your fitness goals.

Within these recipes, you also gained helpful information on how to prepare for a workout. It's important to fuel the body before intense training, but during a specific time frame. Certain foods will give the right kinds of energy for your workout and allow your body to work as efficiently as possible. Remember to always stay hydrated and to properly replenish the body afterwards.

We hope you enjoy these recipes. Making small moderations to meals you already love will give your body the fuel it needs while allowing you to remain on a vegan diet. Remember that these recipes can always be adjusted to reduce or increase macros. Meal planning, prepping, and leftovers should help you get through your week with limited temptations, since these dishes are sure to satisfy.

Whether you're embarking on this journey alone or with family/friends, we hope that you'll spread the message that you can be the healthiest, strongest version of yourself while on a vegan diet. We thank you for taking the time to read this book and wish you nothing but success on your bodybuilding fitness goals! Please leave a kind review if you've enjoyed this book and found any information helpful, and visit our website http://simonarau.me for additional information and bonus material!

References

Drewnowski, A., & Rehm, C. D. (2013, May 28). Sodium intakes of US children and adults from foods and beverages by location of origin and by specific food source. Retrieved from https://www.ncbi.nlm.nih.gov/pmc/articles/PMC3725 480/#!po=39.473

Battaglia Richi, E., Baumer, B., Conrad, B., Darioli, R., Schmid, A., & Keller, U. (2015). Health Risks Associated with Meat Consumption: A Review of Epidemiological Studies. Retrieved from https://www.ncbi.nlm.nih.gov/pubmed/26780279

Caspero, A. (2014). Protein and the Athlete - How Much Do You Need? Retrieved from https://www.eatright.org/fitness/sports-and-performance/fueling-your-workout/protein-and-the-athlete

Florio, G. M. (2015, April 16). 5 Ways Animal Agriculture Is Destroying The Planet. Retrieved from https://www.bustle.com/articles/76177-5-ways-animal-agriculture-is-destroying-our-environment-because-consuming-animal-products-has-a-very-real

Greenfield, B. (2017, February 22). Sports Nutrition 237: How Much Fat Can We Absorb Per Meal? Plus:

'Ideal' Meal Frequency and Supplements For Strength and Endurance Competitions. Retrieved from https://www.enduranceplanet.com/sports-nutrition-237-how-much-fat-can-we-absorb-ideal-meal-frequency-supplements-for-strength-endurance-competitions/

Jeukendrup, A. E. (2011). Nutrition for endurance sports: marathon, triathlon, and road cycling. Retrieved from https://www.ncbi.nlm.nih.gov/pubmed/21916794

Keegan, K.(Producer), & Anderson, K. (Director). (2017). What the Health [Video file]. Retrieved from https://www.netflix.com/

Key facts and findings. (n.d.). Retrieved from http://www.fao.org/news/story/en/item/197623/icode/

Kroenke, C., Kwan, M.,Sweeney, C., Castillo, A., Caan, B., High- and Low-Fat Dairy Intake, Recurrence, and Mortality After Breast Cancer Diagnosis, JNCI: Journal of the National Cancer Institute, Volume 105, Issue 9, 1 May 2013, Pages 616–623, https://doi.org/10.1093/jnci/djt027

Life-cycle analysis study suggests eating less meat. (2019, March 19). Retrieved from https://www.foodengineeringmag.com/articles/89503-life-cycle-analysis-study-suggests-eating-less-meat

Milken Institute Study: Chronic Disease Costs U.S. Economy More Than $1 Trillion Annually: Keeping Education ACTIVE: Partnership to Fight Chronic Disease. (n.d.). Retrievedfromhttps://www.fightchronicdisease.org/latest-news/milken-institute-study-chronic-disease-costs-us-economy-more-1-trillion-annually

Mohr, C., & R.d. (2019, December 3). How Much Protein Can Your Muscles Absorb In One Sitting? Retrieved from https://www.menshealth.com/nutrition/a19525156/how-much-protein-can-your-muscles-absorb/

New Study: Cut Your Carbon Footprint by Going Vegan. (2014, July 2). Retrieved from https://mercyforanimals.org/new-study-cut-your-carbon-footprint-by-going-vegan

Preiato, D. (2019, November 19). A Vegan Bodybuilding Diet: Guide and Meal Plan. Retrieved from https://www.healthline.com/nutrition/vegan-bodybuilding-diet#method

Prostate Cancer. (n.d.). Retrieved from https://www.pcrm.org/health-topics/prostate-cancer

Q&A on the carcinogenicity of the consumption of red meat and processed meat. (2016, May 17). Retrieved from https://www.who.int/features/qa/cancer-red-meat/en/

Q&A on the carcinogenicity of the consumption of red meat and processed meat. (2016, May 17). Retrieved from https://www.who.int/features/qa/cancer-red-meat/en/

Sci-Mx. (2019, August 5). SCI-MX. Retrieved from https://www.sci-mx.co.uk/blog/many-calories-bodybuilder-eat/

Seufert, V., Ramankutty, N., & Foley, J. A. (2012, April 25). Comparing the yields of organic and conventional agriculture. Retrieved from https://www.nature.com/articles/nature11069

Streit, L. (2018, September 27). Micronutrients: Types, Functions, Benefits, and More. Retrieved from https://www.healthline.com/nutrition/micronutrients#benefits

What About Protein: The Science on Protein. (n.d.). Retrieved from https://gamechangersmovie.com/food/protein/